M000012943

WITHIN

Within

Karen Diaz, RD

**Making Peace with Food and
Body Image to Create a Healthy
Family and Home**

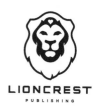

LIONCREST
PUBLISHING

COPYRIGHT © 2018 KAREN DIAZ

All rights reserved.

WITHIN

*Making Peace with Food and Body Image to
Create a Healthy Family and Home*

ISBN   978-1-5445-1277-8 *Paperback*
   978-1-5445-1276-1 *Ebook*

To all the muses in my life:

Julio, the muse of limitless devotion and belief

Claire, the muse of kindness and strength

Lucas, the muse of passion and laughter

To all women who show up so their children see

the strength in struggle, even when they doubt

themselves. You are the muse of bravery and love.

Contents

Introduction

"It's too late for me. Save her."

Many women who suffer from eating/body image disorders feel they are beyond the point of overcoming them. They suffer in silence as they work, take care of the home, and raise their children. They don't realize they are passing on the same food and diet beliefs and concerns to their daughters until, suddenly, the daughter is now a teenager with her own disorder.

That's where I come in. As a registered dietitian certified in intuitive eating, I use my expertise to guide people in overcoming their disordered eating and body image issues. Not just teens but also their mothers, because it's never too late to get started. You can absolutely have a healthy relationship with food and provide a healthy environment for your family. This book will show you how.

A NEED FOR BALANCE

I've wanted to work with women who struggle with eating disorders since I was in high school. My best friend battled anorexia, and I struggled with my inability to help her. I shied away, and our friendship ended. When I went off to college, I discovered that one of my freshman-year roommates was bulimic. I continued to find myself surrounded by women with eating disorders, and something in my heart told me to get a degree in nutrition so that I could better serve them.

During college, I realized my major didn't quite cover the areas on which I wanted to focus. My coursework centered more on food service and food science rather than psychology and eating disorders. In fact, I would estimate that approximately 50 percent of the dietitians in my program had issues with food, and soon, I fell into the same trap. I became obsessed with food and counting calories. I thought, *I'm a dietitian and need to eat perfectly to be a poster child for healthy nutrition.* In reality, I was miserable and had low energy. Thoughts of food consumed my mind, and I realized there had to be a balance.

When I graduated from college, I found it difficult to land an internship or job working with women who struggled with eating disorders. I spent three years gaining experience in pediatrics, food allergies, and weight management at the University of Medicine and Dentistry of

New Jersey and Mount Sinai Hospital in New York. My husband was offered a job across the country, and we were preparing to move when I learned about a position running a nutrition program at the Renfrew Center, a residential eating disorder clinic in northern New Jersey. I had no directly relevant experience, but I knew I needed the job. I walked into the clinic and told them I was meant for the position and would do whatever it took to succeed in it. They hired me, and my family canceled the move.

I worked with women of all ages but spent most of my time with teenagers, teaching them how to manage their disorders. They would successfully leave the program but often encountered problems when they returned home. I had taught them to be balanced and relaxed around food and to not use food as an outlet for their emotions, but some of their mothers' practices around eating often made this difficult. In many cases, these mothers suffered from their own disorders. They would eat different meals from the rest of their families or eat at different times than they did. The mother would weigh herself daily after I had told the daughter to remove any scales from the home. I truly felt sad knowing these mothers were obsessing about food and their weight when, in fact, I knew they could turn it around, feel calm around food, and feel more confident in themselves and own their worth.

I saw it time and time again: women who had struggled

with food issues for thirty years and felt they had no chance of overcoming them. I knew I was meant to serve these women. As much as I loved working with teens, my focus moved to helping their mothers. I wanted to give these women confidence and joy and show them that in eight to twelve weeks, they could have a personal shift and also a shift in the home. They could teach their children that they could overcome something they'd long struggled with.

You can, too. This book is the perfect place to start that journey.

PEACE WITHIN AND PEACE IN THE HOME

I've separated the book into two sections: *Peace Within* and *Peace in the Home*.

Peace Within is dedicated to you. It is designed to help you explore your relationship with food and your body, as well as work on your feelings of self-worth. Do you deprive yourself of food that you love? Are you obsessed with the diet culture? Do you appreciate your body? Do you feel you need to look a certain way or be a certain weight in order to be happy? Do you feel worthy, and do your actions align with that sentiment? These are just a few of the questions we will address and work through in the first section of this book.

Peace in the Home deals with creating a positive home environment, having proactive conversations, and establishing healthy mindsets. You will assess your family values and learn how to bring that to the dinner table. I will walk you through how to reenvision meal time and how to keep food *neutral*—a concept that doesn't define food as good or bad but instead asks that you notice your body and how you feel when eating.

To truly find peace within and in the home, you must first understand what healthy eating and body image look like.

LIVING YOUR HEALTHIEST LIFE

I have a manifesto for women that showcases how I define mental and physical health:

We believe...

Fear tactics don't sway us to follow a certain diet.

We deserve to feel satisfied with our food and life.

Personal happiness is essential.

To be selfless, you need to meet your needs first.

In giving everything to things that bring us joy.

There's no room for apologies in cutting
out things that drain energy.

In living for the present moment without
guilt of the past or worry of the future.

Fear should not paralyze. We use fear
as a guide to help navigate life.

We strive to look in the mirror without shame.

We have quieted the voices saying we are not enough.

We are enough right here, right now. It is not
superficial to want to lose weight, but self-
love in the present is crucial to acceptance.

The perfect diet is eating what looks
good, tastes good, and feels good.

We follow our own path for health with confidence.

We accept that what works for one does not work for all.

We embrace imperfections and highlight strength.

We are free. The light inside of us shines bright.

I share this manifesto and use it as motivation with all of my clients. We continue to reflect on it as we work through their food and body image disorders.

One of the first things I teach is that there are many different ways to eat healthy. You may meet someone who follows a paleo, vegan, keto, vegetarian, or clean-eating diet. If they chose this diet because it aligns with their ethical and moral values and makes their body feel amazing, chances are, it was easy for them to implement and they've remained excited about following it. If they follow the diet because they hate their body, want to lose weight, or were told by someone to give it a try, chances are, they were not as excited about implementing the diet and are less likely to achieve their goals.

I don't subscribe to any particular diet plan. I don't believe there is a perfect way to eat, and there's no plan that fits every human. It's more important to look at the why of food choices. Do they fit with your lifestyle and morals? Does the food provide you with energy and mental clarity? Does it taste good and leave you feeling satiated? Any given diet plan may not work until you can actually get healthy with food and choose the plan from a proper frame of reference. This requires figuring out what matters to you first so you're not swayed by anyone else's input or diet suggestions.

I've seen several cases where health and dietary choices don't always coincide.

Right out of college, I served as an intern at New York Presbyterian Hospital. One of my rotations was in the cancer unit, and I remember my excitement one day as I prepared to meet with a new patient to discuss antioxidants and how food could help her fight cancer. I dressed in my cap and mask, but as soon as I stepped inside her room, she told me to get out. I told her my name and that I was her dietitian, but she didn't care. She said, "I did everything they told me. I ate at local farms, I ate organic, I didn't eat any meat. I did all of this, and I still got cancer. Get out of my room."

This honestly changed my life because I realized so many people have beliefs surrounding their health and nutrition that aren't necessarily true. It's unfair to think a particular diet or way of eating will keep you cancer-free; rather, it's best to learn what works for you individually and focus on health in general.

A recent client learned at a routine exam that her blood pressure was too high. She was scared—legitimately scared. She didn't like how her high blood pressure made her feel, she didn't want to be on medication her whole life, and she was nervous about her future. Her doctor suggested that she lose weight, but I suggested otherwise. The goal was to lower her blood pressure, not the number on the scale. She could make broader changes to her diet and activity to lower the blood pressure, and she would most likely see other health benefits as well. Even if her weight stayed the same, if those numbers improved, she would not feel like a failure.

Food certainly matters and can serve as medicine, but it doesn't necessarily cure everything. Neither does the number on the scale.

THE EMOTIONAL IMPACTS OF DIETING

As I mentioned above, if you do whatever it takes to lose weight, that loss will not be sustainable.

It may feel great at first. Friends may tell you that you look amazing. Meanwhile, you'll feel exhausted and hungry because you allowed yourself only an apple and a protein bar that day. The focus becomes about how you can control yourself to manipulate your body, and everything else falls to the wayside: the nutrition density of the food, your energy levels, your enjoyment of the food, and even your willpower. You will suddenly find yourself at the grocery store purchasing ice cream, only to start a cycle of guilt for having binged. Weight cycling—having your weight go up and down, up and down—has more health risks associated with it than maintaining a level of weight your doctor considers too high. My goal is to have you feel desensitized to food so that the next time you walk down the ice cream aisle, you say to yourself, "I'm good."

Your weight can only regulate once you get on the path to health. You need to let go of the number on the scale and make changes to your eating habits that positively impact your energy levels and overall physical and emotional well-being.

EMBRACING WHAT YOU HAVE

A variety of experts have provided evidence that your body has a "set point" weight. Based on biological conditions, this is a stable body weight that your body maintains with little effort. You have energy and focus, are able to be active during the day, and can still eat food that tastes good in moderation. Your body will fight to stay at this set point weight, even if you head to the gym every day. Reaching a different desired physique will require a maintenance plan to lose or gain weight. If you don't enjoy investing that time, your body will most likely settle back to the set point.

Beyond the set point weight, we all have different body shapes and types. No matter your weight, that shape is not going to change. If you're pear-shaped, you're going to be pear-shaped even if you lose fifty pounds. Your legs and butt will still be larger than your bust. It's time to accept your shape. If you have curves, wear a wrap dress and heels. If you have a smaller chest, throw on a pair of skinny jeans and a tube top. If you are pear-shaped, try an empire-waist flowing skirt. Instead of focusing on what you *can't* wear, focus on what you *can* wear.

If you're not sure what looks best, consider hiring someone to assist you. Several years ago, I sent my measurements, hair and skin color, and photos of myself to a stylist. She put together a Pinterest board of clothing styles that she called *Classic Chic*. My confidence grew and my stress lessened because now I knew exactly how to shop. I didn't get sidetracked by cute bohemian shirts that looked amazing but would never suit my personality or body type. Instead, I looked for the pencil skirts, jackets, and V-neck tops my stylist recommended. There is a style that looks amazing on you that someone who is a different shape couldn't pull off.

Feeling good about yourself means accepting your weight and body shape. But it also requires a shift in how you perceive others. Women of all body types envy one another for various reasons. I've sat in a room with women who range in size from a double zero to sixteen, and the size double zero has said to the size sixteen, "I wish I could share my emotions like you. I'm so scared of everything, and I let everybody overpower me. I feel like I have no voice, and you speak your mind so freely." And then the woman who's a size sixteen would respond, "I wish I had your control. I feel like I put myself out there so much, and I get judged and feel hurt. I feel things so deeply that it's painful, and it makes me want to eat."

These women both have amazing traits that others envy. It's time to embrace what you have and let that shine.

REFRAMING THE QUESTION

When it comes to a healthy body image, we need to start asking different questions. Instead of thinking, *How am I going to lose the weight?* it's time to think, *How can I have more energy? How can I better take care of myself? How can I love myself more? How can I feel more relaxed around food?*

This book is meant to be a framework for you to create positive experiences, establish a healthy relationship with food, and trust that you're making the right decisions because they will now align with your personal, family, and spiritual values. You will identify your values and your vision in Chapter One. These will create a solid base for any future decisions surrounding food and exercise. You will be able to have honest conversations about food and body image, and goals will no longer be tied to a number on the scale.

I created this book to inspire conversations among women suffering from eating and body image disorders, and to normalize discussions on this topic. You're not alone. So many people struggle with feelings of shame, guilt, and fear. They feel isolated and unsupported. Reaching out to others is a demonstration of strength. Disordered eating shouldn't cause someone to feel uncomfortable. We can work through the disorder and get to the other side. We don't have to pass our eating disorders on to the next generation.

These chapters incorporate worksheets to help you put to use the concepts you'll learn. Remember, this book is split into two parts—one devoted to the work within and one devoted to the work with your family. But no matter what kind of work you're doing, it's always critical to trust what speaks to you. If a concept doesn't resonate with you, move on to the next chapter. While I've ordered the chapters of each part of this book in the way I believe will be the most helpful, I encourage you to trust that you're going to read what you need to read at the right time.

Just as there is flexibility in how you view this material, also know there is flexibility with yourself and how you view food and health. People change. Who you are today is not who you're going to be in ten years, and the worksheets may yield different results if you revisit them in the future. The fundamental concepts will still be relevant.

All you need to do is give yourself that grace to be able to shift as you change.

Let's get started!

PART ONE

—

Within Yourself

CHAPTER ONE

Establishing the Framework

The first step in the journey toward finding peace with food and body image is to truly accept the goal of health over weight loss. Most people don't recognize that a number on the scale is not directly a reflection of their health. They want to have peace with themselves. They don't want the chaos around food or to obsess about each bite they put in their mouths. When they come to me and follow the plan I set forth, they see results. They no longer obsess about food, they sleep better, they crave sugar less than before, and they stop bingeing. But often, if they don't attain a magical, toned, perfect body, they think they've failed.

That's what we've been sold as a society. Eat healthily and everything changes. Don't get me wrong: you may love going to the gym, lifting weights, and attending classes. You may want to challenge yourself in fitness, but know that it won't necessarily guarantee you will look like an ideal you were sold on. Everyone's body is different, and the critical step is to realize you're worthy of being happy, having fun, dressing nice, and feeling sexy—no matter what the scale says.

CHANGING YOUR FOCUS

Imagine that your daughter is meant to be a size ten. Do you want her to spend her entire life starving herself, avoiding nourishing foods, and trying to fight her body? No. This applies to boys as well. They may feel pressure to appear muscular to show they work hard or to feel safe from bullies. You wouldn't want that, so why do you want that for yourself? Why do you tie your self-worth to your weight? Why is your happiness based on a number or fitting into a pair of jeans?

Food and body image struggles lead some people to alcohol, bad relationships, or a poor relationship with money. Let go of the idea that you need to look a certain way and be a certain size to be happy, because that concept will permeate your whole life. Instead of, "I need to be here in order to feel X," rearrange your mindset to say, "I want to feel X, so what do I need to do?"

How do you shift your goal from weight loss to being healthy? Expand on the idea of how you want to feel. Adjust your mindset to keep it focused on your destination.

In the past, you've probably stepped on a scale and envisioned that when you lost the weight, you would finally feel at peace. That you would feel calm, accepted, loved, and worthy. But the key is determining how you can feel those things now. *Today*. You need to love yourself to heal. If you're meant to lose weight, you will through that place of feeling peace, calm, love, and worthiness beginning now. When you intentionally delay experiencing those feelings, you do this through a place of deprivation, pain, and sacrifice, and you remain in a place of feeling empty, disconnected, and unloved. Even if you achieve some of your physical goals, these feelings will continue to have a negative effect on your frame of mind and impede your larger journey toward overall health and well-being.

If someone has a million dollars in the bank, the money alone will not make them happy. In order to enjoy it, they need to tie their fortune to a larger purpose. I know that I want freedom, to travel, and to donate to charities. That is how I feel empowered, loved, and connected. It's what I *do* with money that makes me feel good about it. It's not the money itself. The scale is in the same realm. You may have an idealized perception of how you'll feel once you hit that goal number, but in reality, your satisfaction and peace will ultimately derive from the larger purpose you connect to your efforts.

REJECT SOCIETAL NORMS

Society still judges those who are overweight. We can't escape the underlying belief that overweight means lazy while a toned physique means happiness and hard work. Whether it's in person or on social media, people continue to make judgments about those they perceive as less than the ideal. The majority of people aren't shaped like the actors on television, but we're not yet to the point of feeling comfortable and embracing diversity as normal.

When people make reference to "being real," it bothers me because a size two is real, a size ten is real, and a size twenty is real. And being a size two doesn't mean the woman loves her body. She might judge her cellulite or dislike her body shape. I have often heard people confess that at the times they were in the best shape, they were the least happy. We can't continue to judge or think someone is healthy based on their clothing size, in either direction. Knowing you are judged as beautiful and feeling pressure to maintain a weight, or being told you need to lose weight by a doctor due to your size without delving into the whole picture can be mentally stressful in either case.

A POUND DOESN'T CHANGE YOU

When I worked at the eating disorder clinic, I used to lead a group of girls over to the scale and weigh myself in front of them. Afterward, I would step off, drink two cups of water, and get back on the scale. The number would have gone up a pound. Had my body changed? Was I different? No. The only thing that had happened was that I drank two cups of water.

I even performed this exercise when I was pregnant and weighed the highest weight of my life. The girls were shocked by the water-weight gain but even more by the fact that I would step on the scale in front of them. I asked them, "But do you look at me any differently now that you know exactly how much I weigh?" Not a single one did.

Think of a time when you were a smaller size. Were you happier then than you are now? Was your life perfect? Was it everything you wanted? Most people can relate to looking back at an old picture of themselves, whether five or ten years ago, and thinking they looked amazing, thin, and pretty. But if they think back to how they felt at the time, they remember that they weren't happy. Maybe they didn't feel great about themselves or wanted a better relationship, or more money. Maybe they wanted to lose weight and now they are thinking they wish they could be that size.

This has happened to me. I am not immune to it; I just have the self-talk to get around it and don't let it linger. When I lived in Costa Rica, I felt terrible about myself because of the humidity. I felt sweaty all the time, pulled my hair into a ponytail, and hardly ever wore makeup. I didn't want to work out and felt stressed because I was financially supporting our family. I gained weight and felt so uncomfortable. It really wasn't the weight that made me uncomfortable. I was simply reacting to a lot of change at once. Recently, I watched a video of myself there and thought I looked awesome. What had I had to complain about? It was a good reminder that our weight and body can become an area of distraction for other things going on.

It's important to challenge this thought process. Avoiding the mirror until we are happy with the way we look can make the discomfort worse and affect our food choices because we are not in a state of acceptance. Truly see yourself through kind eyes, not critical eyes. Instead of looking back and seeing your beauty, feel it now. Look in the mirror and say, "I am beautiful. People love me. I have a purpose. I give back. I help people. I have a place in this world, and just because I'm picking myself apart in the mirror right now doesn't mean that's what's true." Get comfortable giving yourself compliments and fully receiving them. Start with one compliment. It gets easier the more you give yourself permission and choose this option. If not feeling good about yourself causes daily suffering, it's a sign you need to take a step back and investigate whether underlying emotional issues are affecting you.

CHANGE YOUR MINDSET TO CHANGE THE GOAL

A diet has an end goal. When you get to a certain weight or size, you can stop dieting. You're able to harness willpower and motivation because of the goal. You endure the pain for the promise of happiness later.

What if you decided to change your mindset? Identify the beliefs and underlying emotions that you are avoiding. From there, you can work on finding new habits that make you feel fulfilled and peaceful now. There is no end date; rather, it becomes a way of living every day.

Diets can be seductive because of that high hope for a better body and life. The lie in that is to say you can't have that right here, today. Allow your best self to shine instead of battling to become something later on. The work involves many steps, but at the end, most say they will never go back to the way they were. They want to retain their new sense of calm with food. They want to release their focus on food and their weight. They want to be comfortable in their skin.

It is scary for people to let go of the weight-loss challenge because they fear that if they do, they will balloon out of control. In reality, however, once someone has shifted their mindset and has started looking at food and their body in a different way, it allows them to change. They can see social media posts and diet ads and not be swayed by them. They get to that place where they can enjoy that turkey sandwich and leave half of it on the plate, or they can opt to skip dessert that day. Food no longer rules their lives, and they can enjoy going for a run in the fresh air. Their focus is no longer about getting in that thirty-minute run because they *have* to get in shape but rather because they enjoy it. They never want to go back to how they were because they love how they feel when they've regained their energy. Would you rather hate your body as you wait to get thin and feel good, or would you rather feel good today, regardless of your size and shape, so you can set goals in your life from a place of love?

LIVING IN THE GRAY

Almost everyone I work with tells me they are a black-and-white person. They're either all in or all out. They're on a diet, or they're out of control. But that's not how you were born. Seeing things in black and white is a trait you can change, and the process of listening to your body and trusting your intuition is not a black-and-white proposition. This is different for everybody, which is why I can't help clients by simply giving them meal plans and telling them what to eat. Theirs is not a nutrition-education problem. It's a mental health and diet-belief problem. And a critical aspect of addressing it is learning to live in and embrace the gray area.

This principle is relevant to various elements of this work, including choices made around food. Martha strictly believed she needed to provide healthy meals for her family and never stray from that goal. One dish she often served was a healthy version of chicken parmesan because her kids wanted it every week. The recipe involved grilled chicken with fat-free mozzarella and whole wheat pasta topped with fat-free marinara sauce. Almost every meal she cooked was a low-calorie, dry version of a classic, but she was losing control and bingeing most days.

We decided to make the regular version of chicken parmesan one day and enjoy it without guilt. She agreed to try the experience. She breaded the chicken and fried it, then topped it with full-fat mozzarella and sauce. On the side was white pasta with regular marinara sauce. The kids were thrilled. Martha admitted she loved it as well. She also felt full faster, ate less of it, and was satisfied all night. Analyzing without judgment, she realized the fried chicken was too heavy for her stomach, and now it was a choice, not a rule, to avoid it. She chooses to feed the family the grilled chicken version, using a low-fat cheese blend, and serves the meat with whole wheat or white pasta depending on her mood. This is a good balance for her, a good gray area. Removing the "what I should do" and "what I have to do" helped her find and celebrate enjoying a meal.

June often made spaghetti for her family. Her thoughts were consumed with needing to lose weight, so she would make spaghetti squash for herself and pasta for her family. She was miserable eating the meal. She felt deprived and jealous watching them enjoy the pasta. She needed to be reminded she was allowed to dine on foods she wanted and had the ability to make those choices. One evening, she decided to have the pasta with her family. After a couple of bites, she started to have stomach pain and felt bloated, so she stopped eating. She ended up making herself the squash and enjoyed it for how it tasted and made her feel. The key is that this decision came from a place of choice, not a place of deprivation. Her body had begun making good choices because it craved feeling good. Now she enjoys the spaghetti squash and has gone on to lose eighty pounds without dieting by making aligned choices with room for flexibility.

Mara felt bad about her body and was told she needed to focus on losing weight because of an autoimmune disorder. Her body was changing with age, and she was not happy. With a family wedding coming up, she was disappointed that her weight had not changed. I always encourage my clients to feel amazing where they are now and to buy clothing that fits them well.

It was time for Mara to go dress shopping, and she bought an outrageous outfit for the wedding. It was very unlike her. She was usually someone who blended into the background, and this outfit was red and flashy. She was so excited that she posted pictures to our online support group. When the day of the wedding turned out sweltering hot, she couldn't wear the dress because it was more of a winter outfit. She pulled another dress that was the complete opposite—simple and casual—from the closet. At the wedding reception, the first thing she spotted was a sign on the wall that said, "Own it, bitch." She took a picture of herself in front of the sign and said it was the most fun she's ever had at a wedding because she wasn't focused on food or clothes, only on people and connecting with family.

CELEBRATE EVERY MILESTONE

I encourage everyone to celebrate their successes and milestones, no matter how small. The sidebar showcases some new ways to judge your progress. Know that you're moving forward, and you can choose how and with whom you celebrate. You can celebrate privately, with your family, with someone reading this book, or even publicly on your Facebook page. It doesn't matter. The key is to celebrate yourself because these milestones are a big deal!

WHICH MILESTONES WILL YOU CELEBRATE?

☐ First day you stop weighing yourself and trust the system

☐ First day you feel free from food thoughts

☐ Unfollow/unsubscribe social media/newsletters that make you feel deprived or less than

☐ First time you notice an urge to binge or emotionally eat and choose to delay reacting (even if you still give in)

☐ First time you leave food on your plate and consciously end a meal

☐ Organize closet and ditch clothes that don't fit or are uncomfortable

☐ First time you schedule a daily routine, stick with it, and reflect on the benefits

☐ Create a vision or ideal day that feels exciting

☐ First time you pre-journal meals and/or batch cook for the week

☐ Eat a meal previously forbidden without feeling guilt and allowing satisfaction

☐ First time saying no or yes to something you normally wouldn't because you are honoring your needs (e.g., going out with friends)

☐ Realize you want to change something in life and take action toward it

☐ Doing something that brings joy and allowing yourself to enjoy the moment

☐ Hear a negative comment and it has no effect or you don't take it personally, and move on

These milestones are a reflection of the progress toward a life of trusting your intuition and body so you never have to overanalyze food again. When you are conditioned to praise yourself for following a meal plan or judge success by the number on the scale decreasing, the transition may feel confusing as you look for ways to know you are moving in the right direction. My hope is that these milestones will offer you peace of mind on the journey.

Choose tokens or events that are special to celebrate completing these milestones. They can be big or small, and completely personal. One person I know celebrated with her first-ever manicure. You may get manicures all the time and not think twice about it, but this was special to her. There was a nurse who wore the same pair of sneakers every day to work for years. She believed it was a waste of money to buy herself a new pair, so her way of celebrating was buying herself some new Skechers. Every time she looked at them, she remembered her progress and felt worthy with the reminder she deserved to be comfortable at work.

Whether anyone shares in your celebration doesn't matter; you just need that moment of celebration for yourself. You might treat yourself to a movie or go on a girls' night out. It's nice to commemorate your milestones because they are a big deal to you. You're committing to a new way of life that's healthier for you and your family.

Shifting your focus from weight loss to being healthy can seem hard, but I believe you have a choice in making the journey easy or hard.

First, define "hard" for yourself. Maybe you've spent your life trying to harness your willpower and restrict your food intake only to give up on yourself and spiral out of control. You judge yourself and say no to social invitations because you're not happy with the way you look. You don't stand up for yourself in relationships with friends or romantic partners because you don't have confidence.

That is hard.

In my view, instilling your new mindset is *not* hard. It might feel confusing, but you're reading this book for a reason. You have a nagging feeling that you are meant for more. You're not meant to live a life bogged down by food, weight struggles, or body image. Listen to that voice and decide that this journey can be easy, because it *can* be easy. Give yourself the confidence to challenge your old mindset. Don't believe every article you read. Trust yourself and your own instincts. If you allow the path to be easy, the shift happens so much faster.

Your past does not define you. It is not your identity unless you choose for it to be. Today, in the present moment, is where you can choose to move forward. When you think an action from yesterday dictates who you are today, it's time to redirect your thoughts and lessen the pain. Pull the lessons you want to learn, then close the door to the past before you make choices today.

Focus forward. Get over that fear of "It's not possible for me." You have to decide that it doesn't need to be hard. You absolutely can choose easy.

As you begin to change your beliefs, those around you may be slower to catch up. This is normal. Instead of using that as a barrier to moving forward, create a new community that can lift you up and encourage you to thrive. Create your own support group of friends and acquaintances who may have been yo-yo dieters, or join ours at The Free Life (http://thefreelife.com). Read this book and talk about it and celebrate together. I once belonged to a Facebook group of moms who posted pictures of their messy houses because they were sick of seeing all the perfect Pinterest pictures. It was hilarious! Create your own environment. When you do this, you'll realize what's normal.

I remember when I sold my house in New Jersey to move to Costa Rica for a year abroad with my family. Many people who meant well would say things like, "What are you running from?" or "If you leave, you won't be able to afford coming back to this area." Even with a strong mindset, I started to doubt myself. Thankfully, a friend reminded me that if I ever felt alone, I could find my tribe. I posted in a huge online business support group asking if anyone had ever wanted to move abroad with kids. After 362 comments, dozens of private messages offering help and encouragement, and new friends I still connect with years later, I realized I was normal. Finding new environments when we are growing and changing is a way to make the journey more enjoyable.

WORKSHEET: SET YOUR VISION FOR THE FUTURE

Exercise: Write out your ideal day—from the moment you wake up until the moment you go to bed. How does it look? How does it feel? Base it on what you want, not what you have. If it means you work from home but you work at an office, so be it. The how is not important now. You can use this to focus on how you want to feel every day and what actions will get you those feelings.

Below is a Mad Libs-style worksheet for you to complete as an example. Use the words in the table to fill in how you want or imagine your life to feel at the end of this journey. (You will also need two positive friends in your life to share the one word they think of when they think of you.)

Read it every day or in times of struggle to remind you of where you are headed and help you let go of the stories of the past.

Calm	Peaceful	Sexy	Loved	Confident	Motivated	Comfortable
Satisfying	Delicious	Happy	Kind	Accomplished	Proud	Fierce
Fabulous	Pretty	Beautiful	Smart	Put Together	Fit	Connected
Restful	In Control					

When I wake up in the morning, I smile as the sun hits my face. My feet hit the floor, and I slip on my soft, caramel-colored slippers and my comfy robe as I head downstairs to the smell of rich coffee. I feel _____ about my day as I enjoy each slow sip before the rest of the house wakes up. I enjoy a _____ meal for breakfast before I head upstairs to get dressed. I choose my favorite outfit and feel _____ as I put it on. I wash my face and fix my hair. I look in the mirror and feel _____ of how far I have come. I never thought I would feel _____ and _____. My day is per usual. I have a _____ lunch with a friend, finish my day, and head home. I make my friends/coworkers feel _____ and _____ [fill in words your friends sent you]. When I walk through the door, I _____ to unwind from my day. As I prepare dinner, I feel _____. The day ends with a _____ meal and I feel _____. Maybe I want a snack later or maybe I don't, but it feels amazing not to be _____. I fall asleep feeling _____.

CHAPTER TWO

—

Letting Go of Emotion

You've established your framework and set your vision. The next step is to learn to identify how you cope with emotions, such as anger, resentment, and jealousy, as these emotions can be signals that teach us the why behind our choices.

Emotional ties to food can be rooted in experiences you had as a child. Let's say dessert was used as a reward. You came to associate that with love and affection, and now, when you're feeling a lack of love, you reach for the cookie jar. Many people use eating—or even starvation—as a way to cope. It may feel like an addiction that needs willpower to overcome, but it is time to challenge that thought.

EMOTIONS AT THE CORE

The struggle with food and body image is a lesson that will help teach you about your feelings. You may think you're weak because you should be able to control your eating. If those are your thoughts, you're missing what your body is actually telling you. Your body wants food for nourishment and to function properly, not to replace an emotion or help you work through a problem.

People still use food for reasons other than nourishment or healthy pleasure. They eat because they're feeling stressed, angry, or sad. This kicks off a downward spiral. They judge their eating behavior and feel guilty. They don't remain present with food, so they eat fast, fail to taste it, and get no satisfaction from it. They suffer a physical reaction because they completely blow past their fullness cues. They then restrict the next meal(s) to make up for their binge. They wonder what is wrong with them and berate themselves for being unable to control themselves instead of recognizing the issue as something they can figure out. The answers are all there when you separate emotions from the food.

REMOVING THE POWER FROM FOOD

So many of us give food too much power. We think a healthy choice will lead to weight loss, or one unhealthy choice might cause cancer. We fail to listen to our bodies because we believe there is so much power behind every bite and every decision we make. In reality, however, there are many factors involved in health, including stress, emotional health, spiritual health. This is why we need to step back and rely on our body's wisdom to tell us what we need.

When we give food too much power, we constantly judge what we're putting in our mouths. We try to consume what we are told will heal us and avoid food we are told will make us sick. Yes, food can be used as medicine and to help soothe ailments, but our health is not determined by one day or one meal. How many times have you heard the story of the runner who always ate healthy but died suddenly from a heart attack? Or the story of the grandmother who ate sweets every day and lived to ninety-nine? Stress and worry don't keep us healthy or happy. Eating should be full of pleasure and be stress-free, regardless of how our plates look.

When you believe the food is stronger than you, your mind may race all day long. Each moment your brain says, "I am not going to eat that" and is constantly testing your willpower. When you finally give in and eat that cookie or brownie or ice cream, your mind calms down. It doesn't have to race anymore because you gave it a break. This was not a willpower problem with food. Part of removing the power from food is taking time to center yourself and calm your overwhelmed brain, not exhausting your will-power with beliefs and systems that don't support what your body needs.

IDENTIFY YOUR EMOTIONAL BAGGAGE

We carry with us the stories that we don't let go of. They can be stories of personal shame, the loss of a loved one, a comment someone made, or a time we were wronged. These stories can get heavy to carry. The mistake in making any changes, food and exercise included, is that we skip the step where we identify the stories, forgive them, and let them go. Holding on to them keeps us in a space of reliving the emotions. It limits our energy resources as we shift into a new way of living. Carrying around these unproductive feelings and allowing them to fester hurts no one except ourselves.

PARENTAL BLAME

One common concern my clients face is anger or frustration in how their parents raised them and how this has resulted in issues with food. One mother locked up food to prevent her child from snacking. Another child was home alone every day after school and turned to food as a source of comfort because she was scared. It would be understandable for these people to blame their parents and think their lives would be better now had those problems not occurred.

Asking the right questions can help us reframe this belief. "Is that true? How do you know your life would be perfect?" If the situation had been different, the assumption is no other problems would have existed. When you are honest with yourself, you know times of strength and growth have come through struggle. Had things been different, your life could have been better, but it also could have been worse. Making assumptions only toward the positive makes resentment harder to let go of. The truth is, without that issue, another worse problem could have surfaced. Empathy and compassion doesn't mean the pain was OK; it means you can heal by seeing through another's eyes. Why did your parents act a certain way? What was their life like growing up? Trust they did the best they could with what they had or knew at the time.

Give your parents credit for the good as well as the bad. You are who you are today because of the lessons they taught you, even the "negative" ones. If your mom was selfish, maybe you learned to be empathetic and take others' feelings into consideration. Regardless of whatever story your parents gave you, you control the choices you make in the present moment. Taking responsibility for what you're doing and where you're going is empowering. You did not have control over how things played out growing up, but now it is yours to own. You have free will. You get to choose who you will become.

Some people can let go of their stories easily and move on. For others, the struggles may go deeper. If you don't feel safe as your issues rise to the surface, I recommend you reach out to a licensed therapist for help. Some people can go through an exercise with me, write it out, release it, and feel better. For others, the task may be far more emotionally draining. As you explore your own deeper-seated issues, be mindful of how much the process is taking out of you and consider whether you need additional support.

SPOUSAL CONCERNS

Expressing feelings of anger or resentment toward a spouse or partner for not helping enough or not showing affection can show up in your food or body story. One woman turned to food instead of having a confrontation with her husband over her needs going unmet. Another binged at the end of each day because she was exhausted from running around and maintaining the home. It can feel easier to avoid discussions with our partners, yet this can lead to shutting down and turning to food for comfort.

When you want to feel accepted, loved, and heard, it is time to go within and decide what part is an internal problem to solve and what part is about communication and asking for help. Let's not assume the other person knows what you need. Self-responsibility is letting go of expectations of how something *should* be and instead accepting it as it is. From this place, you can decide where you have control to change the routine and where you can ask for help.

There are always options. We are not victims. In fact, I know you know just how powerful you are. The first five years of my marriage, my husband was off at work, out with friends, going sailing, and playing soccer. It seemed he would do anything to be out of the house, and I was angry because I wanted him to want to be home more. I became more angry and lonely the more I asked him to be home and spend time with us. The more I wanted it, the more he resisted. I dug deep and decided to find what I needed within. I took responsibility for my own happiness. I started a business. I made more playdates with moms. I went out for fun without him. I started to feel fulfilled and enjoyed the times when he was out of the house. The result was, he wanted to be home more. He saw the shift in me, and it shifted something inside of him. Even if he hadn't changed, I had made the choice to still be happy. The answer was inside of me all along. It is for you as well.

CONSTANT COMPARISON

If you face jealousy and constant comparison with friends, turn it into a positive force.

Elisa always said, "I have this friend who always looks perfect and dresses to the nines. She's always in shape and eats whatever she wants, and I wish I could be like her." In this case, I asked her to shift her focus. Why was she drawn to that person? Was it her confidence? Was she accomplished and challenging herself to learn things? Was she well-connected because she put herself out there? Typically, jealousy is about something internal that you need to cultivate and draw out.

Remember, you don't always know what's going on behind closed doors. At the eating disorder clinic, we had women of all ages and sizes sitting around doubting themselves and wishing they were like others in the room. They said things such as, "I wish I had your control. I wish I could light up a room like you and make everyone feel happy." Maybe your friend doesn't eat dessert, but when she goes home, does she have a good relationship with her husband? What's going on in her family and in her head? Do you want that person's life, their whole life? My guess is no. When you think of trading lives—not just bodies—you start to realize all the amazing things you'd be forced to give up, because you can't have just their body and keep your life. You love your own life, so love who you are and the body you live in that helped create it.

Working in the clinic made me more empathetic, which in turn allowed me to live a calmer life. I remember I went into lunch at the center one day and one girl became very upset over a comment I made. She still felt rage from a fight she'd had with her mother the night before. Because I was there representing the food she needed to eat, her anger turned toward me. "I want to throw this plate at your head," she said. I didn't take it personally. I knew the back-story that led up to that comment, and we worked through it. Later that day, I went to Whole Foods to pick up dinner, and a man was yelling at the cashier in frustration about the wait. Usually, I would think to myself that he was being rude, but I had thought back to the girl at the clinic. What had happened to this man that led up to that moment that he exploded and yelled at the cashier? I didn't know his story. His behavior wasn't necessarily acceptable, but I was able to handle the situation with love and compassion.

Do the same for yourself.

STOPPING THE CYCLE

When there is a lack of trust in our body to guide us, we fail to make decisions based on the present moment. Choices are rooted in living in reactions from our past or deciding the future before it happens. Let's say you ended up snacking late last night out of boredom, so you decide you need to start the day with a healthy break-fast—or no breakfast—because you feel bloated and this is the only time you can control yourself. The days get too hectic and you are starving, so you end up making choices you prefer to avoid as the afternoon progresses, stopping for fast food or snacking from the break room all day. Your breakfast was decided based on guilt about the night before and making up for more emotional eating later in the day that hasn't even happened yet. You predict the afternoon will derail and it most likely will. You've already given permission for it to happen. Then at night, this pattern might lead to bingeing, emotional eating, not feeling satisfied, guilt, or shame. You say you will make up for it the next day, and the cycle repeats.

In order to step out of this cycle, you may need to take two weeks and plan timed meals that are not necessarily based on hunger. Schedule three meals that include a carbohydrate, fat, and protein without going more than five or six hours in-between. Have a healthy snack if you go longer than six hours—one that includes a combination of two macronutrients (carbohydrate, fat, or protein). While this may sound counterintuitive to tuning into your body signals of hunger and fullness, it will help you step out of the cycle. Your current pattern means your body doesn't trust you. You can't say you don't like breakfast when you are basing it off late-night eating. To start recognizing the pattern your body needs, break the cycle with timed meals for a few days or up to two weeks. Then start making choices based on how you feel in the present without deciding how you will act later.

Remember, some emotional eating *can* be normal,

healthy behavior. We all have birthday cake at a party or ice cream with friends. Many of society's messages say, "Stop emotional eating!" But it's vital to keep in mind that there's a difference between emotional eating as a constant habit and normal, healthy emotional eating that helps us connect with people around us. Getting ice cream with a friend when you had a tough day is not something to avoid as it can be a positive experience. Eating it every night and feeling you can't avoid it without finishing the container feels different.

ASSESS YOUR TRIGGERS

Julie had four kids and a job she loved. She was a guru in her business, and clients loved her. She underwent a lot of spiritual healing to deal with her weight and body image. She stopped bingeing, got her food cravings under control, and began to dress to suit her body type. One day, she called me. She had been feeling so great, so she stepped on the scale. The number hadn't decreased as much as she thought. She couldn't believe it. She felt so deflated. *What's the point?* she wondered. I asked her what made her step on the scale. If she felt so great and had let go of the idea of tying her happiness to a number on the scale, why did she do it? That's a form of self-sabotage. Something else had to be going on outside of her normal routine.

Julie told me her husband had left for an overnight business meeting. Whenever he wasn't home and she was alone with the four kids, she had a lot of anxiety, and that caused her to binge. The body will get what it needs because it is used to the pattern of soothing anxiety with food. She was approaching a situation where she usually binged but had stopped the behavior. Stepping on the scale gave her the reason she needed to give in.

I asked Julie, "What can you do instead?" She said she could call her husband and tell him how she felt. She did, and they ended up having a great conversation. He calmed her down, and she was able to get the focus off the weight and get back on track. If she had not identified her anxiety and redirected herself away from eating, she would have been trapped in that thought process of "I'm never going to change. This is what I always do."

When you fight willpower, the fight exhausts you. It depletes your energy until you have nothing left. When you're exhausted, you make emotional decisions, and this makes it much easier to fall into patterns. When you embrace your struggles as opportunities for learning, however, you will feel peace because there is another answer. Then you can calm down and listen.

When you look at eating as something you're doing wrong, it triggers feelings of shame and brokenness. When you start fighting the urge to eat, the effort depletes your willpower and energy. But when you embrace the urge, it can give you a positive benefit. There is a lesson your mind is eager to learn. Find it. Listen to what your body is saying to you so you can figure out how eating is helping you cope, and you can replace any unwanted behavior tied to food with a positive, healing behavior. You will start to feel grateful for your body's mechanisms and clues.

When we can find that positivity and gratitude and look at things in a different way, we don't have to feel ashamed anymore. We can harness our intuition and knowledge and everything that we've been through to figure out this puzzle.

Nancy recently took a trip to Italy. She returned and felt like she had completely wasted the trip because the entire time, she was bingeing and purging. I asked, "Look, did you have fun during the day?" She said she definitely had. She had gone on tours and seen the beauty of the country. She'd eaten amazing food but binged and purged at night. This is what she'd chosen to focus on—her memory that ruined the trip.

As we discussed this, I told Nancy that the bingeing and purging was her coping skill. It wasn't healthy, but it had actually helped her enjoy her trip to Italy. It had calmed her anxiety. It wasn't a coping skill she wants to continue to rely on, but having relied on it in Italy did not mean she'd wasted the trip.

This applies to you as well. Even if you have struggled with food and body for years, life still happened. Lots of beauty was born in your life. Find it. Remember it. You are ready to let go now; celebrate that.

RELEASE THE OUTCOME

Disordered eating has a positive purpose. If it didn't, you wouldn't be doing it. It may not be the coping skill you would choose, but it's the one your body developed, whether it was rooted in your genetics, environment, or what you were taught. Everyone's body has a way of speaking to them. For some it is bad relationships, alcohol, overspending, or feeling angry all the time. Your struggle is something you can figure out when you see it through this lens.

Your task is to find the positive benefits of your disordered eating—meaning, how it helps you cope. When you feel the urge to eat, stop and assess whether you're in a heightened emotional state. If you are and you want to feel calmer, pause and consider what nonfood-centered activities would get you there? Come up with a list of activities you can engage in to achieve your desired feeling-state. If your goal is to feel calm, perhaps you can listen to soothing music or an inspirational podcast. Take a nap or a hot shower. If you feel lonely, perhaps you can call a friend or go out to a coffee shop and be surrounded by people. Consider the different heightened emotional states that may cause you to look to food for comfort and come up with a list of five nonfood-centered activities you can test and experiment with.

If you feel anxious and do nothing more than allow yourself to sit with that feeling, take some deep breaths and delay eating; this is a step forward—a progress milestone to celebrate. Delay is success. Release the outcome of what happens after. You can eat the cookies. You can binge. You can emotionally eat. Those methods are always options. Don't decide that success means if you delay, you can't binge or eat. This can cause a rebel effect where the urge is stronger because you've told yourself no. Give yourself space and then reassess the urge when the time is right, knowing you can choose the food if you want. And even if you eat after, if you have delayed your choice, you have taken some power out of food.

Changing your mindset won't happen overnight. Tolerating emotions and finding other ways to handle them doesn't automatically eliminate the urge to use food to cope. If you were learning to swim and I threw you out in the middle of the lake without a life jacket on, you would just flail around. Learning to swim is a gradual process. Sometimes, you will need the life jacket. Think of the emotional eating binges as a life jacket. You may need it for a time. The key is to release yourself from the feeling that you have somehow failed if you do and move forward with kindness toward yourself. When you learn to release the outcome, the results of this work happen even faster.

APPRECIATIVE LOOKING

I once did a photo shoot with Wendy Yalom, a photographer I adore (she did the cover for this book).

I had never felt comfortable in front of the camera, and I wanted to experience what that felt like—to just let go and feel really beautiful in the photography session. I wanted it as a way to help my clients. So many of them avoid photos because of how they look, but I want their children to have memories of them *now*, not only once they feel they've achieved a certain look.

I hired Wendy for an eight-hour shoot. She has a way of talking to you and telling you how beautiful and amazing you are. I felt incredible all day long. I didn't think about anything—how my stomach was sticking out or whether I had a double chin. Afterward, she told me that when I saw the photographs, I wasn't allowed to ask her to alter anything. I had to go through all of the pictures three times, and each time, I had to find one thing I liked about every photograph. She called this appreciative looking.

When I saw the photographs for the first time, I didn't feel so amazing, as she suspected might happen. But I did what she said. I went through 190 photographs three times and chose what I liked about each one. By the time I finished that process, I didn't ask her to fix or touch up any of them, except to iron out one wrinkled dress. It changed my life because I got to walk the walk.

It's still a choice every day. We're all women with insecurities. These exercises are not in vain. We need to do the work to feel good about ourselves. I now have my clients go through old photographs three times and do the same thing. I want them to really push themselves to find different things to appreciate each time.

WORKSHEET: THINK LIKE A SCIENTIST

In order to separate emotions from food, try thinking like a scientist. A scientist wants a specific outcome but has to take an educated guess on how they will arrive there. They create an experiment around the desired outcome and test it. If they don't achieve the results they want, they don't get upset. They don't blame themselves. They don't cry or tell themselves they've failed. They simply look for another way. They adjust and tweak the experiment and try again.

To think like a scientist, you need to take all of the emotion out of this work. When you encounter a negative emotion, look at it through the eyes of a scientist and ask yourself the following questions:

1. Is this true? What would I change about this?
2. What else is going on besides food? (Examine the whole day.)
3. What's different from my normal routine?

Brainstorm alternative behaviors and choose one. See where this takes you and write up a conclusion. Perhaps you'll use the behavior again, or perhaps it didn't work for you and you can try another one. Think like a scientist.

Example:

Every afternoon, Betty craved a cookie from the cafeteria. It bothered her because she felt she couldn't go a day without it. She couldn't identify an emotion tied to the craving, so she decided to test a few theories. First, she thought maybe she was really hungry and brought an apple with cheese for a snack. After she ate the snack, she still wanted the cookie. Next, she wondered if she was bored at her desk and needed a walk outside. She tried the activity but still wanted the cookie. Last, she wondered if she craved social interactions. She went to talk to some coworkers. No more craving. Turns out when she went to the cafeteria, she enjoyed the people-watching and friendly faces she saw. The cookie was just her reason to go. Can you see how if her emotions let her believe she had a sugar addiction she would have missed this lesson? Now it is your turn to put on your scientist hat.

....

....

....

....

....

CHAPTER THREE

Shedding Diet Culture

To be successful in the journey toward making peace with food and body image, it's important to focus on health and balance, despite messages from marketing and society. To achieve this, you need to create a diet-free zone and shed the diet culture.

Shedding the diet culture means making a conscious decision to change your perspective and take a different approach. It means deciding that your life will no longer be defined by a diet. It also means making the choice to change your environment. If you've spent years as a dieter, your environment supports that: your food, your kitchen, your social media presence, your books, even the shows you watch. Is your freezer stocked with frozen Weight Watchers and Lean Cuisine meals? Are your drawers filled with measuring cups and scales (and I don't mean just for cooking)? Is the content you follow on social media related to different diets you've tried over the years? Do inspirational fitness models make you feel less than enough? Does your environment remind you of all the times you've failed at diets or felt out of control?

To transition to an environment that makes you feel calm, you need to embrace a new way of life. Listen to your body and tune into it. Decide that you can trust your body, even if you've experienced ten, twenty, or thirty years of feeling out of control. When you give up dieting, you regain a connection to, and an innate trust in, yourself.

The diet culture looks different for everybody, and shedding it means deleting what triggers you. You may find you're triggered by grilled chicken because it was a staple in every diet you've ever tried. This may prompt a sense of deprivation, which means you should stay clear of grilled chicken while you're working through this journey. Once your mind shifts, you may decide you like the taste of grilled chicken and it makes you feel good, but for now, it's time to stay clear of any triggers and eradicate the diet culture from your cupboards, your closet, and your online world.

FEEL COMFORTABLE TODAY

I want you to feel amazing—*today*. You can't wait until tomorrow to feel good in the clothes you wear. You need to put on things that make you feel comfortable, confident, put together, worthy, and deserving, and you need to feel that now.

Some people hang on to clothes that are too small because they figure they're on the path to losing weight and don't want to buy a bigger size. The problem is, they put on these too-small clothes and feel horrible. That is the opposite of motivation. Nobody ever says, "My stomach is hanging over my pants. Let me take care of myself and eat a nice, healthy stir-fry and drink some water." Instead, the internal dialogue is self-defeating and perpetuates the cycle of dieting or bingeing.

When my clients don't want to invest in new clothes, I encourage them to try clothes through a rental service, such as Le Tote or Gwynnie Bee. They feel pampered, like they're getting a gift every week, all while wearing different types of clothes they don't have to commit to buying.

I also have my clients go through their closet without looking in a mirror. The goal is to put on clothing, dance around, and ask themselves how it feels on their body. If they feel confident and comfortable, then they can look in the mirror and assess. Those comfortable clothes should be front and center in the closet. The rest can be cleared out, put away, or donated. Also, keep accessories readily available. Scarves, earrings, and necklaces—all of those extra things matter in terms of making you feel amazing, today.

These are great methods for the fitting room, too, since you may need to buy some new staple pieces to round out your closet after cleansing the space.

REASSESS SOCIAL MEDIA

Another key step for shedding the diet culture is to unfollow those social media accounts that make you feel judged, unworthy, like a failure, or unaccepted. The owner of the account may be very well-intentioned. More than likely, they don't know you and won't be offended by the unfollow. Examples include specific diet recipe accounts you follow, inspirational fitness models, and exercise programs. Unsubscribe from any email newsletters that remind you of things you feel you've failed at or things you should do and haven't been doing. They may be helping a lot of people. They're just not helping you.

Now it's time to find new people to flood your feed. Follow people of different sizes so you can experience body diversity—women who wear a size ten, fourteen, or twenty and are comfortable in a bathing suit. People can be healthy at a range of sizes. They're not bingeing or emotionally eating, and they exercise and take care of themselves. The more we expose ourselves to the concept of healthy bodies—no matter the size—the more normal it becomes to us.

The body positive space can have an undertone of judgment because supporters and influencers view this as an excuse to give up or not take care of their own body. It is part of the resistance to the belief we have been fed that being thin or a certain size is healthy, regardless of how we get there. Consider unfollowing those accounts that say they practice body love, yet show up without care for their health. This is about what lights you up and feels good to you.

Following role models is crucial because those who embody the healthy lifestyle make you feel really good. We're all on journeys to be the best version of ourselves we can be. It's OK to want a little bit of what your role models have, especially when it's not food or body related. Perhaps you love traveling or crafting. A mom may be passionate about vaccines, and you are, too, so you love how you feel accepted around that. Those are the kinds of internal qualities that excite you. I invite my clients to write down five "buckets" that excite them. The five buckets for me are travel, science, cooking, experiences with my children, and business tips. Find your buckets and follow accounts that post on these topics.

In the beginning, you'll need to experiment with what

feels good, what gives you energy, and what offers confidence. As you develop trust and confidence in yourself, you won't be affected as much by outside influences. I find that when people finally put food in its place, they end up saying they never want to go back to where they were, and that will include those social media accounts you used to follow.

GET RID OF THE GUILT

Maria had been working with me for months. She was progressing well, felt calmer around food, and was finding ways to cope instead of binge. One day, a coworker came in and began gushing over watching the documentary *What the Health*. She had been incredibly inspired by it and decided to become vegan. She urged Maria to watch the documentary and become vegan, too. Maria went home, watched the documentary, and then felt guilty for not deciding to become vegan. Her decision also instigated an almost-daily discussion at work, with her colleague encouraging Maria to make the change. The conflict was taking up a lot of her thoughts and time.

I sat down with Maria and we talked through her concerns. She had tried to eat vegetarian at one point, but her body didn't react well to the diet and she had little energy. However, after watching the documentary, Maria worried she would be hurting her body and acting irresponsibly toward her children if she continued to eat meat and feed it to her family. Maria felt guilty, and as she thought about this further, she realized that for her, it was OK to eat the meat of animals sourced from local farms where they had been humanely treated. Maria also understood that documentaries are designed to be emotional and to provide only that evidence that supports their conclusion. We all have the right to research, ask ourselves questions, and agree or disagree with others' conclusions.

THE CRITICAL-THINKING LENS

Assessing everything we see, read, and hear through a critical-thinking lens begins with understanding that not everything is exactly as it seems. Various types of evidence can support all kinds of ideas and theories—in some cases, conflicting ones. I once sat in the waiting room of a car repair shop. I glanced at the television and saw a newscaster cutting into a piece of steak. The caption at the bottom of the screen said, "Atkins diet lowers our risk of heart disease." Many people argue that a diet high in animal meat and fat is not healthy, but this particular report was claiming the diet was actually good for your heart.

The volume was low, so I moved closer to listen. I looked up the study the reporter was referring to only to discover something very different. The diet the study claimed was good for heart health was heavily plant-based and included moderate levels of carbohydrates from various sources such as sweet potatoes and lentils. It was *not* the Atkins diet. It wasn't high steak, high meat, or high animal fat. But if you only looked at the news and saw that headline and video clip, you would most likely come to a different conclusion.

I always ask my clients to do their research and even take it one step further. If you see an article that says deodorant causes breast cancer, and it's a very emotionally charged article aimed at selling all-natural deodorant, explore it. Click on the study it refers to, read it, and perhaps you'll discover that half of the people in the study didn't even wear deodorant and got breast cancer. Perhaps you'll discover that the researchers were legally prohibited from testing breast cancer tissues, only healthy tissues, and that in reality, there wasn't a strong correlation between the use of the deodorant and cancer.

By researching deeper into a topic, you will see the source and the possible motivation behind the results. You can still decide to buy the all-natural deodorant or eat the steak. But you will be basing this decision on facts, not emotion. You may not care if the study is inaccurate; if it costs you nothing to switch deodorants and you would ultimately feel better about using fewer chemicals, you can make that good, well-thought-out decision. But if you constantly feel swayed by the media or your colleagues or if you feel pressured to change your behavior, know that it might make sense to take a step back and look at matters through a critical-thinking lens.

When you build your foundation with rock instead of sand, you won't be swayed emotionally by everything you read or see. You will know what works for you and what is healthy for you. When you don't know what you stand for, you fall for everything. Developing a critical-thinking lens is not just about reading something and believing it's true and you need to do it. You must consider whether it really works for you.

DON'T HATE THE DIET CULTURE

Shedding diet culture doesn't necessarily mean hating diet culture. I don't believe we should take the stance of us against the diet world—Diet Wars! I don't believe Weight Watchers was created from a negative place. Some people without a disordered relationship with food have followed Weight Watchers and found success and a balance.

Instead of obsessing or hating, it's about coming to a place of calm and neutrality. The weight-loss companies can do whatever they want and it won't affect us. Hating them or turning against them will only serve to bring another level of stress to your life. You must protect your energy and be stronger than the energy of other influences out there.

Often, my clients will go through a phase in which they earnestly reject diet culture, sometimes to the point that they won't even order a salad. They order the cheeseburger just to prove that they can have the cheeseburger, not because it is what they truly desire as a choice that tastes good and feels good. You don't have to eat it to prove that you can have it. You don't have to apologize for eating a salad with your salmon. If it tastes good and you don't feel deprived, then that was what you're supposed to eat. Hating the diet culture leads to rebellion in the opposite direction, and that's not our goal. We are simply shedding the diet culture and not giving it place in our lives.

Once we stop demonizing food and diets, we are released from its impact and hold. But first, we have to set a healthy foundation and develop the trust and confidence that we are doing the right thing.

Place your focus on satisfaction, not deprivation. I show my clients that with all the diets they've tried over the years, surely there were pieces of those diets that worked. Perhaps they loved a morning shake with fruits and kale, or they found that eating a larger lunch and a light dinner worked for their energy levels. I urge them to take a look and determine what felt good to them. As they do that, the cravings start to drop and they feel more satisfied.

For me, intermittent fasting works really well, and I feel good when I sit down and don't multitask during meals. I enjoy those breaks every day. Pay attention to what makes you feel your best and enjoy the foods you choose. Build a new belief system around health and satisfaction, as we will discuss in the next chapter.

WORKSHEET: SHEDDING THE DIET CULTURE

Use this checklist to shed your diet culture:

- Unfollow people on social media who make you feel less than.
- Unsubscribe to all old diets, meals plans, and exercise programs that made you feel deprived.
- Replace foods associated with diet or deprivation in your mind.
- Follow people of different sizes and shapes who inspire you.
- Read articles or watch news that light you up.
- Buy books that are body positive to have around the house.
- Find role models and mentors who are comfortable with food and their bodies.
- Commit to eliminating negative body talk, talking about needing to diet, and/or stepping on the scale daily.

CHAPTER FOUR

Increasing Satisfaction

How we are in life is how we are with food. When you're satisfied with food, you're satisfied with life, and vice versa. Making a change to feel more satisfied on either side will have a positive effect on the other. When your energy feels renewed from less focus on food, you suddenly want to launch the business you delayed. Start taking time to have fun with your friends again, and the role of food becomes less important. When you take time to eat foods that satisfy your taste buds and make you feel good without guilt, then your thoughts are free from food. This new confidence to realize you aren't a food addict can empower you to start to remember goals you left behind or forgot about completely.

Once you have established a mental framework and removed triggers from your environment, it's time to focus on developing a healthier relationship with food.

You do this by focusing less on body image and weight as a result of every food choice. This will allow you to make the right choices in the present moment based on two questions: Will it taste good, and will it make you feel good? Your answers help you live in the gray instead of the black and white.

Want to feel more connected to the gray? Try this exercise: Go online and pull up a menu from your favorite restaurant or one you eat at frequently. Pick the diet option that you would eat when you are trying to be "good." Now pick the option you would eat if you just went off the diet and decided to splurge and be "bad." Now that you have the black-and-white version, find the gray. What meal would taste good *and* make you feel good? What is this in-between meal?

As you shift your focus away from attaining a certain shape or size, you will find it easier to make these choices daily. The inner peace you crave is going to come from building a foundation that supports a healthy relationship with food and your body. From this place, you'll develop a plan you can follow for the rest of your life. If you think of food only in terms of how it will change your body—for better or worse—any changes you make to your relationship with food will be temporary. As soon as you hit your goal, your focus will be gone. You'll return to old patterns and keep yourself in that never-ending loop. Yo-yo dieters have typically been on so many diets, each with a different set of rules, that the rules continue to build into a never-ending pile of contradictions. They get to a point of believing, "Don't eat past 7:00 p.m. Carbs are bad. Fats are bad. Salt is bad. Chemicals are bad." Even though they may follow just one system at any given time, they've accumulated so many rules that they can't let go of them. Following these becomes a confusing, jumbled mess. Right now, identify any rules that don't serve you and release them. It's exhausting to continue to carry them with you.

I'll say it again: your focus must be on what tastes good and what makes you feel good. People mistakenly believe that if they're allowed to have anything at all, they will *always* choose the cheeseburger or the dessert. Is that really true? Would you feel good if you ate pancakes for breakfast, a cheeseburger for lunch, and chicken parmesan with garlic bread for dinner? Would you choose never to have a single fruit or vegetable? Would you choose soda over water every time? Satisfaction is not always based on taste. That's why I pair the two together—taste good and feel good. The truth is, you can have **anything**. If you truly embrace this, you'll find that you naturally crave things in balance. You'll feel less deprived.

Think about non-American cultures whose populations have normal relationships with food and generally aren't overweight. It is not the specific diets, eating at different times of day, or consuming foods native to the culture that prevent these cultures from having an obesity epidemic. Rather, they view food as connection and restful, so they don't experience stress around eating meals. These are joyful moments for them. Americans, on the other hand, tend to be stressed at mealtime, whether it's because of a disorder with food, eating on the run, eating at their desk, or a general dissatisfaction with meal choices.

Something needs to change to quiet the noise and allow us to reconnect.

REPLACE OLD DIET RULES

Moving toward satisfaction means identifying and letting go of any old rules you may have developed so that you can replace them with new mantras.

ASSESS YOUR RULES

Look at each rule individually and decide whether it makes sense and works for you. The goal is to make sure you're not following rules because someone told you to, or because you think there's a right and wrong way to live. It's always nice to have a set of rules that are important to you that support your life and align with what you believe ethically and morally, and that make you happy.

Let's say you chose not to eat after 7:00 p.m. For some, this may work fine. Others may not get home from work until then, or not be able to share dinner with their family until 7:45 p.m. If you have a vision of eating dinner as a family, not eating after 7:00 p.m. is a rule that obviously won't work for you. Holding on to it only causes unnecessary guilt and shame. If you punish yourself with negative talk for breaking a system you set up, this is my declaration for you: step up and make new mantras that work for your life.

CREATE NEW BELIEFS

Once you've identified your old rules, it's time to create new values that are not tied to diets. Examples include I love the body I have; I love the body I was born to have; I choose to question what I hear in society that makes me lose trust in myself.

Once you create these new beliefs, they will perpetuate. If you find yourself watching a news report or documentary, or reading a blog post or book that causes you to question your decisions or priorities, you can glance at your mantras and remember your beliefs. Question the media you're encountering and get back on track.

FOCUS ON MINDFUL EATING

Mindful eating is being present with a meal, savoring all aspects of the food, and removing judgment to experience it while you stay in tune with your body. Mindful eating involves choosing not to multitask during meals. Enjoy the experience while leaving emotions from the day behind you. It will allow you to feel satisfied with the food you put on your plate.

Mindful eating every day, every meal can be challenging and is not realistic for many. I have found there are simple ways to bring this into daily practice that don't take up extra time yet still allow you to slow down.

Start the meal by expressing gratitude or take thirty seconds of silence for prayer or meditation. Depending on which feels better to you, say a prayer to give thanks and allow the meal to be a spiritual experience, or express gratitude for how the meal got on the plate. Think about all who contributed—from the farmers to the grocery store to those who cooked the meal. Ask your children to participate by sharing how they think the food got to their plate. This is a simple way to let go of any stress you are experiencing and become present and focused.

Take the first minute of a meal and eat in silence. Look at the food on your plate and just acknowledge the facts of the meal: "I have a turkey sandwich with lettuce and tomato and a side of coleslaw." For the first bite or two, chew slowly and enjoy your food. Describe how the food tastes to you or have your family describe it. Use descriptive words such as *crunchy*, *salty*, *sweet*, *savory*, and *spicy*.

Leave a bite of food on your plate. This powerful act naturally compels you to be more mindful because it goes against the instinct to clean your plate. Leaving this bite may seem simple, but it is anything but. It may bring up emotions; this is normal. Just remember how powerful this one step can be. Leaving food on your plate not only allows you to be more present at a meal, but it also empowers you to choose when the meal ends. Diets encourage cleaning the plate to get in your allotted calories for the meal. When you go off the diet, the only thing stopping you is your stomach hurting. This is a good reminder to be thankful that our body gives us the gift of fullness. Throw that bite out with gusto and feel the power you just reclaimed: "I choose when the meal ends."

ADD SIMPLE LUXURIES

Luxury doesn't have to mean fur coats and expensive cars. Simple luxuries can completely transform your experience of meals, and making use of them doesn't need to take a lot of extra time or cost a lot of money. Try drinking water from a crystal goblet or drinking coffee from a mug with an inspirational quote. Serve food on beautiful dishware or fold cloth napkins on the table. These simple shifts can make a meal special. It's a way to interrupt your usual pattern and bring you back to the present to really enjoy your meal.

Be creative with your luxuries, especially when it comes to food choices. For some people, it might mean garnishing a plate with fresh herbs, serving fancy mustard, or holding out for a special dessert. You know what your ultimate luxuries are. I especially love key lime pie, anything with caramel, and red velvet cake. So when chocolate, coffee-flavored tiramisu, or cheesecake are offered, I'm not tempted. I know it's worth having the dishes that taste the most amazing to me, so I wait until the next time they are available.

Not only available but *perfect*.

I don't want a subpar key lime pie. I want it to have a nice, crisp graham cracker crust. I want it made with real key lime so it's tart; a pie baked with bottled lime juice won't do. I can absolutely taste the difference. You should establish these luxuries for yourself. That way, it's not, "I can't have this red velvet cupcake because I need to lose weight." Instead, the dialogue shifts to, "Is it worthy of me? Is it worthy of satisfying me? Is it a luxury?" The next time you look at a store-bought birthday cake, you will pass because it's just not worthy of you.

It's time to start getting a little bit pickier about the things you put in your mouth so you know what you are worthy of. This will make you feel more in control, satisfied, excited about food, and supported in life instead of your life being in a frenzy around food.

I will never forget Carrie. She could not stop snacking at night. "I snack and snack. I eat the whole box. I can't stop." She was eating organic cinnamon graham crackers that she claimed she loved. By the time we were done working on her relationship with food and her body, she realized she never liked those crackers. She had cut out and denied herself so many things that she was confused about what she even liked anymore. Trying to follow the diet rules she accumulated over the years, she had convinced herself that she didn't feel guilty over these crackers. She thought they were a healthy pleasure, so she kept eating them, never acknowledging the confusion of why she never felt satisfied. Years of dieting can cause you to think something is enjoyable when it really isn't.

I want you to avoid that trap. Now it's your turn to sort out the rules.

Diet Beliefs to Challenge
- Carbohydrates make me fat.
- Anything with more than x grams of fat is bad.

- Don't eat after 7:00 p.m.
- I am a sugar addict. I must avoid it or I lose control.
- Dessert is only allowed after a healthy meal or eating your vegetables.
- Fasting will help me lose weight.
- I can never eat a white food.
- Skinny foods make you skinny.
- The answer to everything is more protein.
- I need to detox.
- I have to skip dessert.
- I have to weigh myself every day to stay on track.
- There is a right and wrong way to eat or exercise.

New Beliefs to Consider

- I eat foods that taste good and make me feel good.
- There is a right way to eat for my body and it may change over time.
- Movement should bring joy and teach me about my body by allowing me to connect more.
- Managing my stress is equally as important as the food on my plate.
- No one meal determines my health destiny.
- I make choices to feel how I want to feel, not based on the number of a scale.

ENOUGH IS ENOUGH

Feeling satisfied is also knowing when to stop eating. We're used to finishing everything on our plates. If you're on a diet, you finish everything because that's all you can have. When you get tired of following the meal plan, you stop paying attention. Suddenly, the food is gone, and you feel completely bloated.

Where is the perfect place to stop? There are three levels of fullness:

- Neutral fullness is when you could eat more, but intellectually, you know that you have eaten enough. You'll feel full for another two to three hours and then need to eat again.
- Comfortable fullness is when you could eat more, you do feel full, and now you could go four or five hours without eating.
- Uncomfortably stuffed is when your stomach hurts and you have to stop. It doesn't matter how good the food is; physically, it's painful. I like to call it Thanksgiving full.

I suggest you aim to focus on neutral or comfortable. When you're first starting out, you may not be as present with your eating. You may find yourself eating fast or zoning out and getting to uncomfortably full before you realize it. Keep working on being more mindful and present, as it's a skill and takes time to develop. As you succeed, you'll have fewer and fewer meals where you end up feeling uncomfortably full. Neutral fullness can bring rise to feelings of worry that you won't get enough food. Remind your body and brain there is always another meal. You can eat more when you feel hungry again. This is normal if you've gone through years of feeling deprived, especially if you were eating enough in terms of quantity, just not substance.

FOCUS ON YOUR FOOD

Eating is not a time to multitask. Katie always read while she ate because it's the only time she could get it in. Once she put the books away, she realized how emotionally attached she was to the experience of reading and eating. The food didn't even taste as good when she wasn't also reading. Reading was a form of self-care for her, but multitasking wasn't; she needed to give herself permission to carve out time elsewhere in her day to read.

When you stop multitasking, you don't lose something; focusing on a single task at a time is another form of self-care and a vital one. I'm not saying you can never watch TV or read again while you eat, but it's about identifying those emotional attachments you may have to eating. Discover the experience of simply eating and focus on that. Give yourself permission to get your needs met in other ways.

It's also key to slow down while you eat. Eating your food in two minutes makes it difficult to determine whether you're full. You may not have twenty or thirty minutes to eat, but even ten to fifteen minutes is a great place to start.

EATING QUICKLY MAY BE A SIGN TO REVIEW TYPES OF HUNGER TO MAKE SURE YOU ARE COMING INTO A MEAL WITHOUT FEELING RAVENOUS:

Planned hunger: When you are heading into a 2:00 p.m. meeting and you eat a snack. You're not feeling hungry, but you don't want to feel ravenous during or after the meeting.

Taste hunger: Eating just for pleasure and tasting to experience the food and not for fullness.

Physical hunger: When your body is letting you know through your stomach, head, mood, or focus that it is time to eat a meal or snack. When your stomach feels empty and you could eat but don't have to is generally a good time for a meal as you will regulate the quantity you need the best. For a dieter, they like this time because they feel in control. Letting yourself get to a place of a growling stomach or feeling light-headed makes control harder and sets you up to make choices you are trying to avoid.

Emotional hunger: Healthy emotional hunger is having an experience with your family and/or a culture, or allowing yourself to have a food to soothe your soul. When it becomes perpetual, hard to control, and the only way you can cope with your emotions, then it's time to apply all of the principles we've discussed in this book.

LEAVE FOOD ON YOUR PLATE

If sometimes you eat your entire meal, sometimes you leave food on your plate, and sometimes you go back for seconds, keep it up! This is all healthy. However, if your meal always ends when all the food is gone or your tummy hurts, then it's time to consider your eating habits. Remember the exercise from mindful eating and leave a bit of food on your plate. Symbolically throwing out one bite of food is one of the most powerful things you can do to be mindful and connect more with your body. Leaving one bite is something you must consciously do so that it keeps you present during mealtime.

Some people may argue that throwing out food is negative. We have homeless people who could use it. (This is a common argument if you were raised to clean your plate because there are starving children in Africa.) This is why I donate a certain amount of profit from my business to a charity called Blessing Bags that feeds local homeless people in my area. I tell people, "I'll feed the homeless. You leave the food on your plate because that food you're throwing away isn't going to feed a homeless person. You're eating more than you need to, and your feeling sick won't help them." Throwing out food empowers you! You get more in touch with your body and are healthier. You're more motivated and will do more to better others' lives. Everybody wins.

By choosing what you put on the plate and by eating less, you begin learning what your portion sizes are. In the future, you might take less of something and not waste it. You start realizing how much your body really needs.

THERE'S ALWAYS MORE

There's no perfect place to end a meal because if you don't eat enough, there's always another meal or snack. Some people need to incorporate snacks into their day; some don't. Some work from home; some work outside of the home. Your eating plan will be dependent on your life, but I promise you, there will always be more food.

That being said, it can be key to plan ahead. Carry a snack with you or keep one in your car in case hunger sneaks up on you while you adjust to these new cues. Allow for flexibility in your life.

As you begin to work on staying present and finding satisfaction, it can be an unpredictable journey some days. Many people avoid their present state because they are uncomfortable and they don't want to face any emotions that creep in. You may feel you are wasting time or don't deserve the time if you carve time out to eat. But being present with your food allows you to assess your needs, your tastes, and your level of fullness. It allows you to access your life rules and diet rules. And it's a skill that takes time to develop.

WORKSHEET: FOOD ROUTINE

There are certain food patterns that support satisfaction and others that support feeling deprived, whether we realize it or not.

Where do your patterns fall?

DEPRIVATION	SATISFACTION
Not preplanning foods and deciding last minute when you are starving	Eating on a plate
	Using a cloth napkin, fancy glass, or nice silverware—simple luxuries
Eating fast (sometimes wondering whether you even enjoyed the meal, because it feels like autopilot)	Saying a prayer or expressing gratitude before a meal
Multitasking and zoning out when you eat	Thinking about the taste, smell, and texture of the food
Picking all day so you never feel full or know whether you're hungry, and it feels automatic	Not taking stress or emotions into a meal, letting them go before you eat
Eating in the car	Leaving food on your plate sometimes
Eating out of containers	Not eating something if it doesn't taste good
Eating in secret or hiding	Asking yourself what will taste good and feel good
Feeling upset or frazzled if someone comes in while you're eating	Preplanning meals for days that are busy or overscheduled
Taking a bite before you finished the first	Not judging feeling full but feeling grateful our bodies tell us when to stop
Not putting your fork down the entire time you eat	Knowing all foods are allowed and you get to choose
Always finishing the meal or eating until it feels uncomfortable	Garnishing your plate or plating food to look appealing
Telling yourself you can't have something instead of asking if you want it	Having meals with loved ones when possible
	Not multitasking at a meal
	Putting your fork down and staying present at meals to check in with your body

Now identify:

Which food routines do you want to change?

....

....

....

Which food routines do you want to embrace?

....

....

....

CHAPTER FIVE

———

Becoming Self-Full

Once you've completed the journey of exploring within, it's time to pivot toward creating a healthier environment for your family. By finding peace within and becoming self-full, you are better prepared to create a positive environment and model a healthy relationship with food for your children.

The reason I started using the word *self-full* is because selfish isn't a word most of us want to be called. We want to feel and be seen as selfless, although it's almost selfish to be selfless, because if you always give away your energy and desires, then you end up running on an empty tank. Being self-full is about being a fully charged battery, a full gas tank, or a full water bottle. Everyone around you receives the overflow of your energy, joy, excitement, and inspiration. When you are completely filled up, you are excited to be present, to do chores, to help your kids with their homework. The important tasks of your daily life become things you *enjoy* versus things you *have to do*.

THE IMPORTANCE OF BOUNDARIES

Love yourself first to love others best. Failing to love yourself negatively affects those closest to you. Setting boundaries is one of the biggest challenges I see, but it's important to learn to say no and set boundaries around the things that don't work so you can get your own needs met instead of being run by everyone else's needs. If you don't set boundaries, you're basically accommodating everyone else's desires.

If you're a people pleaser, consider how you appear to others when you don't set boundaries. You try to show that you want to care for others, but it has the opposite effect. You become overwhelmed by your obligations and have to back out of them, so you appear wishy-washy. You do a poor job because you don't have time, and this makes you look like you don't care. You get annoyed with yourself for taking on too much, so you become short with those around you. People aren't able to rely on you. This is the opposite of who you are.

This is why it's important to set boundaries and make choices that will fulfill you. Assess who in your life lifts your energy and who drains it. Determine the tasks you have to do versus what you want to do. Doing this will help you begin to set boundaries in your life.

When people know where you stand and what's important to you, it's easier for them to interact with you. They feel more comfortable because they know you have established boundaries. They know that if you say yes to an obligation, you will fulfill it on time and to the best of your ability. I don't want someone to help me and then feel resentful or act annoyed that they have to be there. If I know somebody will tell me if they're unavailable to help me, that sets me free to find the right person. I know I can always ask the person who will be honest with me and tell me where she stands. A yes means she's all in.

It can be challenging to shift to this mindset, but play a little role reversal. Think back to the last time someone failed to fulfill a commitment they'd made and how you felt, or to the last time someone was grumpy performing a task they'd agreed to do. You don't want to be that person.

This topic may uncover a worry that someone won't love you if you don't give to them like you always have. You may derive validation from feeling needed. It is OK to recognize these feelings; just make sure to ask yourself the right questions. Instead of, "Will they love me?" ask, "Do I want to do this? Does this work for me?" This way, you either feel amazing about offering the help or can set your family or friend free to find another solution with love. Those who love you want you to be happy, whether you choose to give or to tell them no.

PRACTICE SELF-CARE

Being self-full matters because when we're in a pattern as moms, we shift our focus to take care of others, especially our family. We let everyone else's needs determine our schedule, and we run in reaction mode, reacting to everything that comes toward us. The end result is that we feel unfulfilled and depleted of energy. We run around on autopilot, busy but without direction. How we are in life is how we are with food, so if you go through life on autopilot and get overwhelmed, you'll go into autopilot with food. Bingeing or numbing out can become your body's way of getting what it needs when you're not choosing another way that is more aligned, healthy, and loving.

Your relationships are a reflection of how you feel about yourself. How do you treat your family when you don't feel filled up? When you get to that point of burnout and your battery is on zero or your gas tank is running on fumes, it's too late because you now need a complete break—perhaps even an entire weekend—to recharge. This isn't always reasonable or doable. Weekends should be a time to enjoy a little time away and various recreational activities, not for recovering from burnout.

SELF-CARE ROUTINES

It's important to practice daily, weekly, and quarterly self-care.

Daily routines keep us present and connected, as well as replete our energy. They are important and the best place to begin. Routines can be thirty seconds, five minutes, twenty minutes, or half an hour. Take ten deep breaths, or throw on a twenty-minute exercise routine. Take time out multiple times a day to clear your head.

Weekly routines can involve lunch with a friend, getting a manicure or blow-out, or taking an afternoon off to read for a couple of hours at a coffee shop. These tend to be longer than the daily sessions and allow time to regroup.

Quarterly routines should involve bigger activities, such as a spa day, heading out for an adventure day with your family, or driving somewhere for a weekend. You need something on the calendar every three months, whether it's with friends or family.

The daily and weekly routines are where you start because that makes the biggest impact in the here and now. My clients know that when you physically exert yourself, such as training for a marathon, it takes time. You have to create a training schedule and put it on your calendar. Sadly, we don't give our minds the same luxury.

We think we should have the energy, focus, and clarity without needing breaks. We know physically, our body will tell us what it needs, but we don't listen to the signals from our exhausted mind. We must choose to listen to our minds as we do our bodies. Take a few minutes to close your eyes, breathe deeply, and give yourself a rest. The mind needs to reset itself. Don't let it get to the point of depletion. Remember, it's much easier to top off the tank than to refill it entirely.

SCHEDULING IS VITAL

I have to have a social event on the calendar each week or I start to feel lonely and disconnected. It can be lunch with a friend, a glass of wine or tea, a phone call with someone who lives far away, or a mom's night out. Be self-aware and think like a scientist. You may need to test your self-care routines. What's the minimum amount that you need to sustain yourself and feel happy and fulfilled? When you know the answer to that, it becomes easier to schedule joy into your calendar.

Prioritize this. Washing dishes does not change your life, and neither will cleaning the counter or doing laundry. It may feel good to have an organized home, but that doesn't move the needle in your happiness. You have to take a stand for your needs. Release the idea that things in your home and life need to be a certain way for you to attend a scheduled event. Perhaps there will be more clutter in your home, but that's not a reason to cancel.

If you've ever been in a moms' group, perhaps you know that the number one thing moms do is cancel. I'm not saying you're never going to cancel, but the event should be rescheduled immediately. Having joy scheduled on the calendar gives you something to look forward to, and it also helps you set your boundaries from an empowered place instead of an apologetic place. Reassess your self-care from time to time. Ensure your choices still work and provide benefits. If you don't check in occasionally, you begin to slip into old patterns and lose the commitment. Get back to your vision and connect it with your practice so that you are making a choice.

Betty was divorced and had fifty-fifty custody of her daughter. On the nights she had her daughter, she felt guilty for going to the gym. She felt she should spend every second with her daughter when they were together. However, when she didn't attend classes or the gym, she found herself tired and frustrated and ended up being short with her daughter. When Betty started going to the gym for an hour, she still carried some guilt, but she felt more excited to come home, put her daughter to bed, and read books to her—a weight lifted from her shoulders.

As a mom, I am not sure the guilt part ever fully goes

away, but you can choose not to use it as an excuse to hold yourself back. Even a year later, Betty had trouble leaving her daughter and going to the gym, but the benefits of her workouts far outweighed the risks associated with her not going. Adding to this, Betty's daughter now had a more present mom and could witness her mother advocating for herself.

IDENTIFY YOUR NEEDS

Participating in self-care requires identifying your needs. To begin, look back on your exercise from Chapter One. Look at the words you put down for your ideal day. What changes or actions do you need to make in order to feel better in these areas? Who do you need to be? All of the necessary qualities are inside you; it's just a matter of bringing them out and giving yourself permission to experiment with them.

Stephany was a receptionist and a mom. She had longed to be an actor and comedian but felt she was too old to pursue that dream anymore. We talked about how to meet that need of acting and comedy so she could feel light on the inside. She found an improv class that she committed to once a week. She hated the first few classes and worried it wasn't the place for her. She felt uncomfortable and didn't like spending the time away from her family. I told her to stick with the class for six weeks. By the time class was over, she loved it. She ended up doing a voice-over audition for radio and TV commercials and signed up for another class. She also found an entirely new community of support and friendship.

When we're used to our routines, we create mental barriers as to why we shouldn't or couldn't do something. We have to stick with the new activity for a while and give it a chance to work.

PRACTICE BOUNDARY SETTING

It's not easy to start setting boundaries, especially if you haven't done it before. The best place to start is to role-play with someone you trust. How do you feel when someone says yes but actually means no? I guarantee it won't make you feel great inside. It's better to say no and understand the reasons why you can or can't do something.

Communicate your boundaries clearly. Passive boundary setting is to say, "I think it might be nice if...," whereas assertive boundary setting is to say, "I want to do X because of Y."

You want to be clear and assertive because not everyone can read your mind and guess your intent. If you're unsure what to say or don't yet know if you can commit, ask for time to respond. This allows you distance and to assess your willingness to commit.

Julie binged on fast food on the way home from work because she was stressed about walking into a dirty house and immediately having to clean. She really wanted a housekeeper but had already decided that her husband wouldn't agree to it. We practiced how she could be assertive in her request. She listed the options and demonstrated how having a housekeeper would allow more time for other activities. "I know that you're busy at work, too, so the best option isn't to have me ask you to do all these tasks. Instead, I would like to try a housekeeper for a couple of months and then decide if it's working or not." This worked better than her saying, "I know it's an expense. And I know it's not what you want to do. But still, I think we can do this, and I'd like to try."

Two things happened. The first was Julie was able to have that conversation and get a part-time housekeeper. The second was that she was able to give herself permission to walk through the door and ignore any housework that might need doing. When I checked in with her a year later, she had stopped bingeing and credits much of that to her new routine when she comes home from work. This involves thirty minutes to herself for a shower, meditation, changing clothes, and leaving the day behind her.

When you set your intentions and know what you want, you start communicating them and everything comes together. Your brain is trained to look for solutions and move in the direction you want to.

WORKSHEET: PRACTICE BOUNDARY SETTING

Pick a scenario in which you need to establish boundaries. Think through a wishy-washy response, and then write out your assertive response. Here are some examples:

Nancy was approached by Heather to join a committee on the PTA for the upcoming father-daughter dance. She is feeling overwhelmed at work but also wants to make more friends and hates saying no.

> Wishy-washy response: "Oh, that sounds great. I would love to. I'll have to check my calendar." (Then I avoid them or spend time justifying why I think I can't as I go back and forth.)

> Assertive, kind response: "Thank you for thinking of me, Heather! Unfortunately, I can't commit and give it what you need. If I think of someone who might be interested, I will send them your way."

A mom calls and asks if you can watch her son because she has a late-night meeting. You are not sure it is a good time for your family but don't want to turn them down if you can do it.

Wishy-washy response: "Of course!" (Then panic that it doesn't work or feel inconvenienced.)

Assertive, kind response: "You know what? Let me call you back in an hour. I just want to check in with my husband and make sure I am not forgetting about any plans. I'll call you at 7:00 p.m."

....

....

....

....

....

....

....

....

PART TWO

—

Beyond Yourself

CHAPTER SIX

Reenvisioning Mealtime

Everyone has a vision of a perfect mealtime. The entire family sits around the table, calm and positive, while enjoying a delicious meal. But how do we achieve that? Through conscious effort—effort that begins with sitting down with your family outside of mealtime and establishing guidelines based on your schedules and shared goals, including connection, nourishment, love, and enjoyment.

CREATE FAMILY GUIDELINES

Family guidelines provide the basis for what mealtime will look like in your home. Every family is different, but the first step to creating the guidelines requires assessing your family values. Once you have defined these, you can then take the steps to support them.

Let's say that you value togetherness and want to share

stories of your day, but your children all have hectic schedules and nobody is home at 6:00 p.m. for dinner. You can adjust your meals accordingly. Perhaps this means a later dinnertime, or maybe you decide that breakfast is the meal you share together.

If your family value is quality time, but you're constantly carpooling or can't find time to squeeze in a daily meal, you could choose to have a weekly meal together. Make it a standing date and break out the china or head to your favorite restaurant.

Look at your values and play with the rhythm that works for your family. You may need to revisit your guidelines on a regular basis because schedules will change. Toddlers need an earlier bedtime, grade schoolers are off and running to after-school activities, and teens may be working, have homework, or a social life! Your family values don't have to change, but the rhythm and schedule and the needs of the kids change. There are many ways to come back to those values, so you will want to reevaluate on an annual basis or on a school-schedule basis.

Once you have assessed your values and built guidelines, mealtime becomes a lot easier to work with. This said, everyone needs to continually make mealtime a priority and make sure it's quality time together. The last thing you want is everyone feeling rushed or trying to run out the door. This means meals don't have to last thirty or sixty minutes. You don't need to fully set the table each night. Connection is the important factor. You can enjoy a meal for ten or fifteen minutes and still feel connected and nourished.

Also, as with all aspects of creating a healthy home and family, give yourself permission to go off schedule. When you've established your guidelines and the family agrees, it's OK to have an off night when something comes up.

AVOID STRESSFUL CONVERSATIONS

Family mealtime is not the time for stressful conversations, whether it's kids talking about problems at school or trouble with a friend at soccer practice, or parents discussing their work. Stressful topics will vary depending on the family, but make a decision to leave those conversations out of dinnertime. The goal is to foster a peaceful, relaxing environment and to facilitate and encourage being present. If we're talking about the past, we're not being present with our food. So keeping dinnertime free of stressful conversation is a good place to start.

You can enjoy silence. You don't have to fill up the time to have a connection, and this is where every family's different. If just sitting and enjoying silence together leaves you wanting more, try some games such as Heads Up or buy a pack of Would You Rather cards. Some families create a jar filled with questions to ask each evening.

Sara Blakely, businesswoman and founder of Spanx, talks about how her dad used to ask her every day, "What did you fail at today?"[1] It always generated a positive conversation at the dinner table, and it showed her that there is always something to celebrate. She credits her current success to that practice of celebrating failure because it means you're moving forward.

GIVE THANKS

There are many ways to stay present during the meal, but an immediate way to bring everyone together and work toward mindfulness is to give thanks or say a prayer. This encourages the entire family to be present. Children may not understand the intention, but gratitude and spiritual practices force them to pause, reflect, and be in the present moment. Your children will understand that feeling of taking a moment to appreciate the process and will carry it with them.

There are other ways to stay present. You can talk positively about the food—about how great it smells or that the plates look pretty. Ask family members to share their

---

1   https://www.inc.com/melanie-curtin/billionaire-ceo-sara-blakely-says-these-7-words-are-best-career-advice-she-ever-got.html

favorite part of the meal. Invite them to think about the texture and taste of the food. This results in mindful eating.

No matter how young they are, get your children involved with meal preparation, setting the table, or cooking when possible. Let them take drink orders from everyone and report back to the chef. Ask them to present the meal to the family before everyone begins eating.

MODEL HEALTHY EATING

Having everyone eat the same meal helps ease the life of the chef and models good eating to the family. It's understandable that some children are picky eaters or have food allergies, but you still get to control the meals. You may serve what you know your child will like and add in one new option of what everyone else is eating. Or you may provide a couple of healthy choices and let them choose what and how much they eat. Praise your child for trying something new.

You can instill the importance of nutrition without food labels of good or bad. We want our children to grow up believing that balanced eating is an important element of self-care and self-love and that food and exercise are not meant to control weight. By providing options that are nourishing and balanced, we can talk positively about food while still giving them freedom to assess what tastes good on their palate. We can control our behavior—meaning making food choices, moving our bodies, and feeding our minds positive fuel. Empower them by focusing on what we can control.

TEACH BALANCE WITH FOOD

Finding balance among a family can be difficult. Some family members may have special dietary concerns that need to be taken into consideration, but it's still important to choose food options that work for the entire family.

DISCREPANCY WITHIN THE FAMILY

When we focus on weight over health, we create a scenario that affects everyone. Let's take a scenario where one child is considered overweight on the growth curve, but the other is not. Jack is a twelve-year-old boy who was told by his doctor to lose weight because his weight and BMI were too high for his height. Jack doesn't love sports and therefore exercises less than his peers. His sister, Sofie, is low on the growth curve and plays a competitive sport. All children need nutrition, regardless of their BMI. Being low on the growth curve doesn't mean nutrition gets thrown out the window, just as being on the high end of the growth curve doesn't mean you never get to eat higher-calorie foods. If you serve them different meals due to their weight, this facilitates the teaching that food and exercise choices are meant to manage weight, rather than to support health. Instead, we need to provide balance and eat foods that nourish our bodies. A discussion around needing more food to support a high level of exercise or having more fruits and vegetables for energy are more than OK. Saying one child can eat a cheeseburger but the other one can't causes food to feel like a reward or punishment based on weight.

I interviewed a mom whose daughter has cystic fibrosis and needs to be at the high end of the BMI scale, so she eats high-calorie foods. But there are also teenagers in the house. We talked about how she models healthy eating for all her children. She had several suggestions for how she manages their balance.

First, she doesn't tell her teens that the high-calorie foods are off limits, because that somehow makes them special. She does explain that this is a prescription of her needs, just like medication would be, so there needs to be enough available just for her toddler.

Second, she gets her teens involved in cooking so they can contribute and make foods that they enjoy. She talks about experimenting with foods so they taste them. This is a special activity she can share with the older children that her toddler can't partake in, so it adds to their bonding.

She used to body bash and yo-yo diet while her teenagers were growing up. Instead of avoiding the topic, she dived in and did the work within. She then talked to them about her accomplishments and about how her ideas on eating and health were passed down to her by her mother when she was growing up. Their new tagline is, "The legacy ends with us."

It's important to teach your kids that sometimes beautiful lessons are passed down to us, and sometimes lessons aren't healthy. You can choose which you carry on and which you choose to end and not pass down. And it is never too late.

MANAGING SNACKS

Jeanne had four children and had struggled with past eating disorders and a yo-yo diet mentality. She was petrified she'd pass her problems on to her children. The kids would come home from school, throw their books on the counter, and raid the pantry because they were starving. She didn't want to limit their choices or tell them they couldn't have the cookies because she didn't want them to end up with her eating issues.

This behavior didn't serve her or them because they were grabbing whatever they wanted, eating out of bags, and not thinking about their food. When dinnertime came, they weren't hungry.

She envisioned the environment she wanted to create and worked on taking the emotion and judgment out of the equation. She realized it didn't make cookies bad if she asked her children that, when they walk in the house, they must put their backpacks away before heading to the pantry. She set rules and boundaries. Her children had to come home, put away their supplies, and then choose from snacks she provided. She laid out chopped vegetables and fruit, sometimes with cookies or chips, but she took advantage of the fact that they were hungry to get in their fruits and vegetables.

Once she told them this plan, she encountered zero resistance because it made it easier for the kids to get their snacks when they were laid out and available.

Because she wanted to decrease stress and resistance, she took a look at what the kids would fight her on every night. It turned out that she had them shower every night, and they wanted to shower in the morning. She agreed to let go of the shower at night as long as they washed their hands and face and brushed their teeth. This way, the kids felt like they were getting something, too. The shifts in routine included things that both she and they wanted.

There's a difference between setting boundaries for your family and connecting cookies with weight problems, and that's an important distinction. It's about teaching them balance and giving them the ability to choose from among options you decide on.

MAKE A PLAN AND WORK IT

Having positive and calm mealtimes often starts with a plan. By planning your meal ahead of time, you know that it will be healthy and balanced and that you won't have to scramble last minute to get it on the table.

Take twenty to thirty minutes to make a basic plan for the week, and you will save yourself time and work later on. I actually take three hours on a Sunday to cook for the upcoming week. I prepare chicken, cook rice, cut vegetables, and store everything in containers. It takes time out of my weekend but saves me exponentially during the week.

If you have an insanely busy schedule, cooking for the week allows the family to sit down and eat together. You can even offer options because the food has been prepared. One person may have tortilla soup one day, and another may have chicken and rice, but they can swap the next day. This is a way to make the cook's life easier if everyone doesn't want to eat the same meal because cooking different meals daily is not sustainable.

You don't need to plan every meal for the week. Leave room for leftovers or takeout. Meal preparation and planning may feel stressful at first, but you can start with simple ideas and build from there. You can repeat the same menu and slowly add in other ideas that can be rotated. Put the menu on paper or on a whiteboard so everyone knows what to expect.

A common argument against food preparation is that you're just adding more to your busy schedule. I say, try it. Try preparing and then take note of how your week goes. Did it save you time, make you feel better, give you less stress, save your energy, and make mealtimes more enjoyable? I promise, you will not feel annoyed, flustered, or frustrated by planning ahead and cooking when you know there are benefits you will reap the following week.

Another recommendation is creating go-to meal ideas and everyday items you always have on hand, especially if you have a busy family and no time to be creative. You can deviate from the plan if something comes up, but most of the time, you eliminate all of the stress and energy expenditure of deciding what to eat in the moment when people are hungry.

Food planning isn't just for dinner. Our family chooses three to five dinner selections, and we also decide breakfast options together as well. We alternate between five options that we vote on when we plan out the week. Whoever gets up first knows the menu for that day and can prepare the breakfast. The entire family has agreed on the options, so breakfast can be quickly put together. You can empower your child to make choices by providing two options, if you'd like. Also, school-aged children can learn to plan in advance to either eat at school or pack a lunch. When packing their own lunch, I recommend going over menu choices and helping them decide what to include.

MAKE MEAL PREP WORK FOR YOU

For those who are creative, you can prepare for more elaborate meals. But for anyone who isn't comfortable with planning, it's OK to keep it simple and experiment. Theme days are an easy way to get started. Taco Tuesday, Soup Wednesday, Crockpot Thursday, Italian Friday, eat out on Saturday. You can vary the recipes, but it helps to easily plan when you work within themes. My family loves the themed menus and looks forward to them. We form memories and make that vital connection.

Jolie hated cooking, but she had a belief that mothers must cook meals from scratch in the kitchen. She never wanted to plan or shop for food, so she delayed preparing dinner, and her entire family felt stressed because they never knew what time dinner would be served or what it would be. She had to work through the belief that it's OK *not* to cook and that there are other ways to contribute as a mother. As she engaged in this process, she was able to model self-care for her children. She had the money to hire someone to cook, which worked for her family.

If you're too busy to prepare meals on your own, you may consider hiring someone to do this for you or look into relatively less expensive options, such as HelloFresh or Blue Apron, from which you can buy premade meals. Or, if you can fit meal prep into your schedule but need to build up your skills, you may decide to take cooking classes. There are also simple recipes available on various online sites or in magazines. I recommend looking for recipes with five ingredients or simple ingredients that you keep on hand. Look on Yummly and save recipes to Pinterest that have limited steps and can be made in a short time. My solution is soups and crockpot recipes, because I can throw the ingredients in and have it cook all day.

Most of all, focus on nutrition, but know that it's OK to mix up your meals. I like serving healthy foods mixed in with the occasional *soul foods*: foods that may not be perfectly balanced but always win in the taste department. Or perhaps you prepare healthy meals at home but let everyone choose their favorite meals at a restaurant. You can even choose to serve pancakes for dinner if you're feeling rushed one day. That's self-care for you and your family and choosing to not always be strict.

WORKSHEET: THE PRE-JOURNAL-YOUR-FOOD CHALLENGE

For one week, determine foods that will make you feel good and taste good.

Breakfast: Three ideas

....

....

....

Lunch: Three ideas

....

....

....

Dinner: Five ideas

....

....

....

....

....

After you execute prepping and batch cooking for one week, reflect on how it went.

How long did it take to batch cook and plan the meals?

How much time did you save during the week?

How did it feel knowing the food was taken care of all week?

What were the benefits?

Would you do it again?

CHAPTER SEVEN

—

Keeping Food Neutral

"You have to eat your vegetables if you want dessert."

Have you heard that before? Have you said it before? It's a very common statement, but I'd like to show you how that approach—and other similar rules—can actually set children up to have negative relationships with food. Instead of labeling things "good" (vegetables, chicken) or "bad" (ice cream, chocolate), I prefer to keep food in the "neutral" category, and I'll show you how to do the same.

Creating this type of environment allows children to tune into their own experience with food. They can determine what is too little or too much or how certain foods make them feel without judgment or rules. They can enjoy all foods while still learning health as the value to hold high. There are no ties to weight or body shape.

A DISCUSSION ABOUT TREATS

My daughter swims with a local team, and we often attend swim meets. At one event, a mom on the opposing team talked to her daughter as she readied to swim. We overheard the mother promise her child that if she beat her own time, she would get an ice cream as a reward. I love the challenge in swimming of competing against yourself and beating your own time, but in our home, you don't have to do something to get a particular food.

I wanted to use this conversation as a discussion point with my daughter. After the meet, we went to lunch, and I asked her if she knew why we don't make ice cream or other desserts a reward for an accomplishment such as a swim time. I explained that we can have ice cream anytime. We don't eat it all the time because it would cause stomach pain, and it doesn't provide us with the best energy. In our home, we decided it is not something to earn by doing a special activity. I asked her how she felt about the two different approaches to open up this discussion and point out that different families have different values.

Having a positive, relaxed view on food helps to limit guilt and judgment. If a food is labeled good, are we good for eating it? On the flip side, if a food is bad, does that make us bad for eating it? Labeling food disconnects our children from their internal cues and natural regulation instead of empowering them. Kids exercise their independence as they become older, and it's natural for them to gravitate toward what is restricted or held back from them.

When you keep food in a neutral zone, it models for your kids what they can control. You empower them instead of giving them rules that generate negative emotional responses. Studies show that you want less of foods labeled healthy and good, and you want more of those that are forbidden.[2] This contributes to a cycle of overeating, guilt, and then restriction.

ENABLE CHOICE

We all know it's important to eat our fruits and vegetables. But we limit the beauty of all the lessons we can learn about ourselves when we eat vegetables solely because someone told us to.

While the intention is good to promote nutrient-rich foods and limit "junk foods," research shows that the more parents try to control or restrict intake, the more children get disconnected from being able to regulate themselves.[3] Being forced to eat something as a child

---

2   https://www.ncbi.nlm.nih.gov/pubmed/10357749/

3   L. L. Birch and J. O. Fisher, "Development of Eating Behaviors among Children and Adolescents," *Pediatrics* 101, no. 3 part 2 (1998): 539-549.

rarely results in your loving that food as an adult. I still don't eat fish because of the time I sat at the table until 9:00 p.m. to finish the fish dinner my mother had served. You don't want to condition your children when their tastes can change later on.

The idea that you need to eat dinner to get dessert conditions kids to believe you have to eat *this* to get *that*, which in turn teaches them that *this* doesn't taste as good as *that*. Try to not attach dessert to being an after-meal treat, or as something you have to eat something else to get. We've even had ice cream for lunch. That doesn't happen often, but if we all want ice cream after a soccer game, I don't insist that we eat a sandwich and salad first. Instead, we choose to have lunch two hours later.

One time, my extended family came together for the holidays. My sister's family had eaten a late lunch and wanted dessert, so we opted to join them before eating our own dinner. The family connection and experience was far more important to me than having dinner before dessert. Nobody is locked into the time of day they must eat meals.

You want your kids to eat their vegetables, but when you put too much emphasis on pushing them to eat certain things, you lose the wider view. Instead of using dessert as a reward, consider experimenting with other ways to fit in nutrient-dense food. Maybe they like fruits and vegetables, but they want different ones than those you are serving. Check by asking them what they want you to buy from the store, or let them physically pick out food. Perhaps they want vegetables raw instead of steamed, or perhaps they want their apple slices served with peanut butter. And it's more than OK not to offer dessert every night. What we are trying to accomplish is letting go of the labels we tend to give foods and not giving desserts so much bargaining power. Invite kids into the conversation to ask how they would like something served or what fruit or vegetable they would like to eat.

Consider making dessert an experience. This is really an important value for my family. I like to visit an amazing bakery to pick out doughnuts with fun toppings, or head to a cupcake store that's known for winning a baking show cook-off. You can even create an experience in your own home by putting out different toppings for a sundae bar. These allow for a family connection to happen around the experience and something besides the sugar to look forward to.

When you adopt a relaxed environment around food, everyone can now make choices without emotions. When your child asks for a treat, you can ask questions in return. Is this going to be the most amazing dessert? Is it what you want to choose, or do you want to wait for something more special? Your confidence will grow as you see they are able to say yes or no because they know the food is not forbidden and they can have it at another time.

CAN WE LOSE CONTROL?

Many adults worry that if they cease labeling or restricting certain foods, there will suddenly be a free-for-all and they'll go for only the junk. They fear they'll eat chocolate all day and never choose to eat a vegetable again.

Mindfulness and intuitive eating have been shown to be more effective than restriction and control. When self-regulation with food and exercise is encouraged and trusted, there is less weight cycling and more peace of mind.[4]

Those who have a normal, healthy relationship with food and believe they can have anything they want when they want it no longer view junk food as special. They even stop craving it all the time. If you prohibit ice cream from your house and never allow your children to have it, they will struggle to limit themselves when it's available. If ice cream is always around, your family will stop focusing on it. None of you will regard it from a place of deprivation or feel you need to eat it all before it's taken away.

---

4   http://www.medicalnewstoday.com/releases/279291.php

After years of yo-yo dieting, an adult may tend to crave forbidden junk foods even more. Reintroducing those foods as something that is now allowed may result in your eating more of it until you can become desensitized and live food-neutral. Children are developmentally different. You don't need to give them so many cakes and cookies that you desensitize them. If you've done the work within yourself, feel relaxed about food and desserts, and incorporate them in balanced moderation, those views will trickle down to your kids. I encourage utilizing a "taste good, feel good" mind frame. Kids understand that language. Something may taste good, but will it feel good? If they ask for chips or candy, ask them, "Is your mouth hungry, or is your stomach hungry?"

Don't worry about those moments when the kids lose control. Halloween and birthdays are great learning tools, because children overdo it and often end up with a stomachache. It teaches intuitive eating. Kids are resilient, and they will learn to listen to their bodies.

LET KIDS BE INVOLVED

There are numerous ways to bring your kids into the food conversation so that they can understand the importance of a healthy relationship with food. The goal is to keep them comfortable around food to support their body and mind:

- Start a garden and learn about growing vegetables. When they get to be part of a project or experiment, they are more invested. They will be proud of growing their own food. You don't need a big yard to get a "grow herbs and vegetable" kit from the store and get started. Once the tomatoes, carrots, or green beans are ready to be picked, let them choose a recipe to prepare the food and taste the fruits of their labor. Having them prep and cook with you will have a much greater impact than reading food labels or being told to eat their vegetables.

- When they try a new food, ask them to describe how it tastes or the texture. Give them descriptive words to choose from. Share how it tastes for you. This is an extension of mindful eating. If they do not like the taste of a food, celebrate trying new foods and always giving something one bite before you decide. Their taste buds will change over time. This way, they will know not liking tomatoes now does not mean later on they won't enjoy them.

- Bring them in on the discussions if you make certain food choices or exercise choices. Instead of letting them interpret what is going on, think out loud. When you are tired and don't want to work out, tell them it is good to rest your body and honor being tired, so mommy isn't going to run today. When you cook salmon while they dine on burgers, talk to them about the special fats you get from salmon and how they help your skin, hair, and energy. Then invite them to taste. Tell them that exercise and food are important to your health, but so are other areas such as sleep, managing stress, and having fun. Take the discussion out of your head and invite them to be a part of it. This kind of talk will help form their beliefs, self-worth, and self-talk when they get older.

· When kids eat something healthy, you can share how proud you are that they take care of their bodies and enjoy foods that give them so much energy. Yet on the flip side, share that you are so happy they enjoyed that cupcake but stopped when they had enough.

We can give our children lessons in health, nutrition, and movement without involving emotions, dieting, and weight. If someone outside of the house comments that their food choice is bad or good, ask your children how they feel about it and then share why you do or don't agree. Ask what they think of what you believe. You will be amazed by their insightfulness and confidence as you give them a voice and allow them to grow.

WORKSHEET: HOW FOOD-NEUTRAL IS MY HOME?

Explore these messages to decide which you may want to show your children. There is additional space to add your own at the bottom.

- Desserts are soul foods to be enjoyed at the highest quality and don't need to follow a meal.
- You don't need to eat or do something to get a treat.
- Food is not a reward or punishment.
- Vegetables and fruits are fun to experiment with.
- There is no good, bad, or forbidden foods. We are a taste good, feel good house.

Additional messages you want to show your children:

....

....

....

....

....

....

....

....

CHAPTER EIGHT

—

Assessing the Bigger Picture

Often, mothers who struggle with eating disorders and body image worry about their children's eating habits and weight. In general, these concerns are more about the mom's fears than the actual health of the children. It's important to look at the bigger picture, both as it relates to the individual child and the entire family.

The bigger picture is about focusing on the things you can control and remembering that one scenario or one choice isn't going to make or break a child for the rest of their life. You have to stop putting so much pressure on yourself. If you say the wrong thing in the moment, if your child has pancakes for dinner, or if your child goes through a period of being underweight or overweight on the growth curve, this doesn't speak to their whole life span. Of course, you love and care about your child and their health. You want to address any concerns with them or their doctor. However, it's important to consider first whether the issue is a persistent and problematic pattern or a temporary set of circumstances.

FOOD IS ONLY ONE PART OF HEALTH

Shawn Achor, author of *The Happiness Advantage* and founder of GoodThink, once spoke to the glass is half-full/half-empty concept. He says, "I would suggest a different way of looking at the metaphorical glass. We get so focused on ourselves and what's inside the glass— our physical possessions, daily moods, failures and triumphs—and we can argue forever about the merits of being an optimist or a pessimist. Ultimately, however, the contents of the glass don't matter; what's more important is to realize there's a pitcher of water nearby. In other words, we have the capacity to refill the glass, or to change our outlook."[5]

If you find you have concerns about your child's weight or eating habits, zoom out and look at the bigger picture. Are they sleeping well? Are they doing well in school? Do they have good friends? Food is only one picture of health.

If you're concerned about choices your child is making,

[5] https://www.success.com/article/is-the-glass-half-empty-or-half-full

just start with a discussion. Ask about school, their friends, and how rehearsal went. Are they physically hungry? Take a look in their lunchbox. Is it empty every time? Perhaps they need a larger lunch. Ask how they are feeling.

Here are two ways to have a simple conversation without labeling food:

- Ask if anything would taste good, or only that particular food. This gives you a guide into whether they are truly hungry (they will eat anything) or whether they are eating as an activity (out of boredom).
- Tell your child that it's time to eat for energy, not taste, so they can focus on homework. "Would you like..." and give two options that are nutritious.

Have these conversations without labeling food. Spinach and kale are healthy, but having a balanced relationship with food is healthier. We want to feed ourselves good food that gives us energy, and we want to feed ourselves good thoughts to make us feel confident about ourselves.

Mental wellness is part of health; we don't want to disconnect our children from their internal cues of hunger and fullness, so it's crucial that we support them. But there remain lifestyle choices that we can control. If you are worried they are forming bad habits and you don't know how to address this, it's time to reach out to a dietitian who specializes in pediatrics for help. It's OK not to have all the answers or to worry that you'll say the wrong thing. You're coming from a place of love.

DETERMINING THE UNDERLYING ISSUES

If your child is eating emotionally or bingeing, not exercising, and their weight is higher as a result, it may be scary to not know what to say or fear you will make them feel worse. Listen. Love. Have empathy. Ask them how they feel. Work with them.

We cannot always see what is going on with our children, but it's not a cause for guilt. Their health is a reflection of something greater going on. Here is an example of a common scenario I would see in my practice, where the parents often found an unexpected solution.

John was a thirteen-year-old boy whose parents were concerned because he had gained weight. They wanted him to learn healthy habits and stop eating sweets and chips in the afternoon. He often sneaked food from the cupboards and hid in the bathroom to eat. When asked how he felt right before he ate, he described a nervous feeling in his stomach, like butterflies, and he said that when he ate, the feeling went away.

It turned out that he felt incredible pressure to perform in sports he didn't love to play. He felt outside pressure to succeed in sports and academics, and this resulted in emotions he didn't understand. He became uncomfortable and turned to food.

Asking open-ended questions allowed John to describe how he felt without judgment. He was able to explore his feelings and determine why he turned to food. His parents thought he needed education on how to live a healthy lifestyle because they didn't recognize there was an underlying reason. The truth was, he didn't want to play sports, and he didn't want to tell his father. All he needed was the courage to say how he felt.

When your child doesn't know how to express their feelings, you can assist by going back to "Thinking like a Scientist" at the end of Chapter Two. Help your child experiment, tune in, and make it fun. This will lead to answers and faster results.

HOW TO SEE THE BIGGER PICTURE

As a parent, there are steps you can take to see the bigger picture in your child's interaction with food. My first instinct is to try to identify any stress or pressure the child might be under. Does something feel off, or has there been a major shift or change in their attitude toward eating? Was the child previously active and now she's fighting it, perhaps by watching TV all the time? What's the environment at home like? What boundaries have you set? Is she going into the pantry without asking or taking food up to her room?

ASSESS ACTIVITY LEVELS

As adults, we may have to schedule thirty minutes of exercise every day to get it in. Children have physical education at school and often participate in sports, sometimes for hours on a weekend if they play in tournaments. On an off day, kids may lounge around reading or watching TV.

Every household is different, but it's normal for kids to be more active at one time and less active at another, and that's OK. That's where you zoom the lens out and consider the bigger picture. If you want them to be more active, consider moving with them! Or create a list of activities they can choose from to see what feels exciting for them.

RECOGNIZE UNHEALTHY BEHAVIORS

Children can absolutely develop unhealthy behaviors around food, and it's important to recognize these. Do you see food in the trash can that you didn't know they ate? Are they going into the pantry without asking? Do they take food to their room? Do they finish all their food and ask for more every time? Do they eat fast? Do they talk about food frequently? Is it difficult to redirect them away from conversations on food? Are they throwing food out and not eating enough? Do they go to the bathroom after meals? Do they say their stomach hurts before or after meals? If you see any of these indicators, it's time to take a closer peek into the root of the behavior in case there is a problem.

If you establish a health boundary and it feels as if your child has an abnormally adverse reaction to it, this could be a sign of an unhealthy emotional attachment or other underlying issues. This is especially true at an older age. It's not a two-year-old throwing a tantrum over a lollipop. A twelve-year-old has enough self-control to manage a tantrum, so if they throw one, that is a sign they may have an unhealthy attachment to the food.

RECOGNIZE HEALTHY BEHAVIORS

The flip side to this is recognizing when your child has a healthy behavior around food and body image. The best way to tell is when you have a conversation at snack time.

Let's say you come home around dinnertime and your daughter is sitting on the couch with a bowl of cheese puffs. When you ask her if she's ready for dinner, she says, "No, I'm eating this."

You know this isn't a healthy option, so you say, "OK, why don't we just save that for your lunch tomorrow, since you won't be hungry for dinner?"

If she responds in the affirmative and puts the bowl away, that's a normal and easy conversation. When raised in a relaxed household around food, children are fine putting a food back because they know it's dinnertime and they can have that snack at some other time.

UNDERSTAND NORMAL PATTERNS

Kids will be kids. Sometimes they want double portions, and sometimes they're not that hungry. Sometimes they eat more adult-sized portions, and sometimes they leave half the food on their plate. This is all normal.

Some parents are concerned that if their child doesn't eat all their dinner, they will want to snack all night. If that happens once in a while, that's fine. If it becomes a pattern, save the dinner and heat it for them later. Or set a boundary and say no snacks. If your child goes to bed hungry, that's OK. She won't wake up malnourished in the morning. You get to establish the rules, but it's also OK if there is a give-and-take.

Remember, not everything is a sign of a bigger problem. If you have a fear related to your body image or food concerns, you may see a small thing in an extreme way and pressure yourself to fix it. That's why you want to recognize such fears and limit or eliminate their power over you. Parents sometimes inadvertently teach the lesson that food and exercise help dictate our shape and size instead of teaching that eating and exercise are tied to loving and caring for ourselves.

CREATE HOUSEHOLD VALUES AND RULES

We feed our bodies healthy food and healthy thoughts, and we engage in healthy movement to stay strong and take care of ourselves. These are acts of self-love and are key for you to demonstrate for your family. Self-love should be a household commitment, led through action and conversation. It should be the basis for your household rules.

But how to start? Look back on your family values and create a simple statement—for example, when we're hungry, we fill ourselves with nourishing foods that give us energy.

Values can change and evolve as kids go through different stages. Defining the values is not about rules. If you don't follow them, it doesn't mean you failed as a family. It's simply about what's important to you and allows you to have a basis and foundation for when conversations and problems arise. Having family values also contributes to a unified stance in the sense that no one is singled out. If you decide to have no soda at dinner, everyone makes that change. Dad can't drink the soda just because he's an adult and you can't control him. That sends mixed messages.

When outside circumstances come up that challenge one of your beliefs, you can have a conversation around this value. Your values and rules can address how you approach sweets or even how you exercise. One family may choose to go to the gym together and talk about the importance of aerobic activity, while another might do yoga and talk about the importance of stretching.

My husband and I decided it was important for our children to each pick a sport to play. My daughter is ten years old and my son is nine. In our opinion, they are too young to know whether they like something or not. They need to try new things and give it time, so we ask that they pick a sport and finish the season. They can opt into a new sport the next year, but it's important for them to learn teamwork and dedication.

My daughter's current sport is swimming. She has wanted to quit at least five times when she got nervous about the meets, but now she loves it and thrives in the pool. It's been a huge boost to her self-confidence and has taught her the value of consistent practice and hard work. Another family might value family activities such as hiking or doing other outdoor activities together. There is no right answer.

ENCOURAGE SELF-AWARENESS

You've heard it before and you'll hear it again: "Mom, I'm hungry. Can I have a snack?"

Whether your child is physically active and needs more food, or whether they had dinner an hour ago or lunch hours ago, your response should be the same, "Why are you hungry right now?"

If it's 8:00 p.m. and your son wants a pretzel like he does every night, it's time to figure out why. Is he eating because he's bored? Is he eating because he wakes up hungry in the middle of the night? He doesn't have to put down the pretzel, but maybe he needs something more nutritious. I always revert to asking, "Is the mouth hungry, or is the stomach hungry?" Another question to ask is, "Will anything solve your hunger, or is it one specific thing?" Typically, if it's one specific thing, the hunger is emotional instead of physical. That's how intuitive eating and listening to your body works. If you don't know whether the hunger is emotional or physical, assume it's physical. You don't want your child to lose trust in their signals, especially if they are being flexible with options presented to them.

We can't control what size or shape we are, but self-awareness is one thing we can control. It's a great skill to develop and to teach our children.

ADDRESS GROWTH STAGES

When children go through puberty, they change in different ways. They may gain weight in their stomach or thighs, or they may have a growth spurt. You don't have control over how they gain weight and fill out. It's inevitable. But you do have control over how you approach these changes.

First, take a look at your family genetics. This is the first clue as to how your children will develop. Have discussions with them about body types and loving your shape and size. Look at those family values and rules, and keep coming back to them. Choose health through the foods you eat and the way you move your body. These habits make you feel good, rather than your size determining how you feel.

Sometimes parents worry how others will view their child,

or they worry about what a doctor will say. You as the parent are the one who sees the bigger picture. When doctors plot your child on the curve, a higher weight for height or BMI should not alarm you. Instead, focus on habits and trends over the years. Not every child should plot on the fiftieth percentile, but there's a fiftieth percentile for a reason: because there's also someone at the tenth and ninetieth on the chart. Be sure you keep that perspective in mind.

Also know that even when you have the best intentions, your children may still develop disorders and bad habits. At the eating disorder clinic, I worked very closely with a family in which the mom was a dietitian. She'd made a point of raising her kids with household rules, and she was rooted in her beliefs. They fueled their bodies with balanced, wholesome foods; they had soul foods in moderation while eating out or traveling. They were quite relaxed around food.

One of her daughters turned out to be a very intuitive eater and had a healthy relationship with food. The other daughter was in treatment for anorexia and dealt with a lot of anxiety and depression.

When I counsel moms who worried they've failed their children, I say to them, "You're a mom who has a child with an eating disorder. You're not a mom who caused your child to have an eating disorder." It's important to remember that despite all your best efforts, there is no way to guarantee that everything will turn out perfectly. This is why it's so important to establish values and a strong foundation. When things don't turn out as you'd hoped or expected, these will empower you and help you remember you did what you could—including, perhaps, seeking out professional help when you and/or your family needed it.

WORKSHEET: CREATE YOUR HOUSEHOLD RULES

Here is my example of our household rules:

The Diaz Family Manifesto

- We believe food is not good or bad, so you are not good or bad depending on what you eat.
- We don't believe you are what you eat. We believe what you eat is a direct reflection of your self-love.
- We believe everyone deserves to live their best life with integrity and truth, so our job as a family is to hold that space for one another.
- We believe our bodies are the home to our souls, our hearts, and our minds.
- We believe dessert should be worthy of us and not a mindless treat.
- We believe foods should taste good and feel good.

- We believe throwing out food is not a waste because we are listening to our bodies, and we give back to the homeless because everyone deserves dignity and respect.
- We believe all emotions are important and should be expressed in a healthy way without judgment.
- We believe we don't need to sit down for a family meal every day, but when we do, it is present and without tech.
- We don't believe food is a reward for a behavior, and we believe some emotional eating is normal.
- We believe in always trying different foods as people change, bodies change, and tastes change.

A manifesto or value system will allow you as a family to come back and remember why you take the actions you take so that when situations of comparison come up, you remember and have a conversation about why you do what you do versus what other families do.

This is your time to create your own family manifesto based on your values. Feel free to borrow any element of mine.

....

....

CHAPTER NINE

——

Talking about Bodies

I believe there aren't enough conversations between adults and children on the topics of bodies and food. These conversations are critical to have. If you feel uncomfortable talking about these topics, remember that every day your children are exposed to other conversations and ideas that may go against your values. Remember, too, that as they age, children go through phases during which they stop listening to their parents and are more influenced by their friends and all media that surrounds them. You can't control how their friends were raised or the content of the advertisements to which your children are exposed, so it's better to establish your influence early.

Shame grows in silence, and that's another reason to have open conversations with your kids. Give them a space where they can reach out for help and feel comfortable talking about their bodies. We want to instill that our body is a vessel, the home to our soul, and we need to treat it with the care it deserves.

TOPICS OF CONVERSATION

There is a variety of topics you can and should discuss with your children.

BODY SIZE

We already established that body size is not something anyone can control. Extreme thinness is not a realistic goal for anyone to strive for, particularly not girls who are going through puberty. A child who is told to lose weight and restricts food to do so will find themselves on a cycle of yo-yo dieting once they reach a weight-loss goal and revert to old eating patterns. Balanced eating—never shame-based—is the key.

Instead, teach your children that we are all born with different bodies, and these are the bodies we are meant to have. Some children will grow tall, some will be short, and their shapes will vary. At different times during puberty, your children will need extra fat for growth and for girls to get their period, resulting in extra belly fat. We cannot control our height or body shape, and we don't want to teach our children that they should try to control things that they can't. What they can control are the food choices that give them more energy and make them feel good. They can make choices about movement, exercise, and sports.

Encourage your children to respect not only diversity beyond culture and backgrounds but also beyond body shapes and sizes. Society may make us feel that having more fat or being a larger size means a person doesn't eat well or exercise. That assumption is not always true, nor is the opposite. A person who is considered skinny isn't necessarily healthy or happy. Empower your child to smile, knowing they can choose happy and healthy and to love the body they were born to have.

WORD CHOICES

Examine word choices and what people do and don't have control over. For example, my son once made a remark about someone being fat. Kids are exposed to that word. When I asked what it meant, my daughter said, "It is an insult, and you shouldn't say it." Even at ten, she was taught that the word was negative and mean.

The underlying message with fat being an insult is the assumption that when someone is a bigger size, they are lazy and don't take care of themselves. Our discussion became about the word *fat* being an insult. I needed to teach them that a person's size can be out of their control. Many people take care of themselves but have more fat on their body or a bigger size than the actors we see on television. It is not enough to simply say, "Fat is not a nice word." The next-level conversation is explaining why it feels like an insult and how we can be part of the change so people can feel more comfortable in their bodies, including us.

SOCIAL MEDIA TRUTHS

Help your children to be media-savvy. As you make your own choices about whom you follow and unfollow on social media, teach your children to do the same. Help them see how advertisers often make people feel bad about themselves in order to sell products. We can't always control what television and movies children see. Choose options featuring different cultures and body types when you can. More importantly, talk to them about marketing. Just like they learn historical trends in school, they can learn that body ideals are trends that have changed over the years. Knowing every person has a body that will work to maintain the right weight for them helps them see why these trends can make us stressed and unhappy.

There currently exists an unrealistic standard of beauty, but things are changing. Educating our children and having these discussions with them are the first steps. Help them develop a sense of identity and learn to value the things they believe in.

TIPS FOR TALKING

When having these discussions with your children, it's important that you keep some key points in mind.

WHEN TO HAVE THE CONVERSATIONS

You'll have times when a discussion on bodies just presents itself, while other times you can decide to bring up a specific topic.

Often, my daughter and I read together at night. I use that time to talk about how I love my arms because I love writing, and I'm grateful I can do that. I ask my daughter what she loves about her body, which leads to a discussion about body parts, how they benefit us, and why we love them. This is part of a quiet time when we reflect on our day.

I keep books around that feature strong, independent girls and women who have all different types of bodies. Favorite books include:

- *Strong Is the New Pretty*: Features kids of various ages along with quotes about what they love about themselves.

- *Good Night Stories for Rebel Girls*: Features bedtime stories about the lives of extraordinary women from the past and the present.

- *Listening to My Body*: This is perfect for younger children, as it introduces them to the idea of paying attention to their body.

- *I Matter (Mindful Mantras)*: Teaches your children to be mindful of their feelings and the world around them.

DON'T PROJECT

I try to stop assuming I know how my children feel and I try to refrain from establishing rules based on my own childhood. Growing up, I wasn't allowed to shave my legs until I was in eighth grade. Perhaps I only remember it this way, but it was how I felt. I was embarrassed and hid in the bathroom while changing for gym class because I didn't want anyone to make fun of my hairy legs. I recently asked my daughter if she had any desire to shave her legs, and she said she loved them as they were. I told her if she changed her mind, I wanted her to let me know. We won't know the exact moment our kids may struggle or have these worries, so be proactive in discussions and open the door for future conversations.

DON'T SHY AWAY

Sometimes kids don't want to engage in certain conversations, but you still need to have them. Ask open-ended questions, buy them a book to read on their own that you've also read, and show them no-judgment conversations are important and safe in your house.

Discussing bodies—our own and others'—normalizes these conversations. Talk to your children about how bodies develop at different times, and that there is no such thing as a perfect body. Ask questions and keep things very casual. Very few parents are comfortable with these topics, but it's important to try. These discussions can make a big difference. Let's choose to let the body image issues end with us.

STAY SELF-AWARE

When talking to your children about bodies, it's important to avoid letting your own fears and issues seep into the conversation. Self-awareness is key. Know that you embarked on this journey to develop a healthy relationship with your body, and that it's a long journey. It's not a magic pill; it's a work in progress. You don't need to be perfect and have a perfectly healthy relationship with food or your body in order to raise a child who has these. Bring them on the journey with you, and let them see that you're proud to be working on what you're helping them learn. This is equally as powerful as demonstrating you've mastered all you're trying to teach them.

My daughter looked at a picture of herself as a baby in which she could see the dark circles she still has under her eyes. These are genetic features from both sides of the family. She said, "I guess I'm always going to have these dark circles." My immediate thought was, *Oh my gosh, she feels bad about herself. She doesn't like the dark circles under her eyes.* But then I realized that she hadn't actually said that. I stopped my internal dialogue and asked her, "What do you think about that?"

She responded, "I love it because when I look in the mirror I see my *abuelita* and my *meema.* I have their eyes."

I said, "You're right. I love that about you."

When you have conversations with your children, continually check in with yourself. Make sure you're not injecting fears, emotions, or assumptions into the dialogue. I find the easiest path to keeping yourself out of the talk is to ask your child questions. Ask how they feel. Ask what they think about a given topic. Then continue from there.

KEEP DISCUSSIONS POSITIVE

Many of us grew up in households where our mothers felt

negatively about their bodies and continually put themselves down. Our own children watch everything we do. They register when we count calories, skip meals, or make comments about not being able to eat something because we need to lose weight.

When you exercise, do you make comments about it being because you ate so bad yesterday or because you want to go out to eat tonight? Don't feel guilty; simply be aware of the messages you are sending your children. You may not ever have the perfect body image, but you can't body bash and then expect your children to exude self-love. You may feel uncomfortable with yourself, but your goal should be to teach your children good lessons and not pass on damaging behavioral patterns.

It takes time, but you can learn to view yourself through a loving lens. Even when it's uncomfortable, this is a skill we want to teach and instill in our children. Children listen and pay attention, and they repeat behaviors they observe. Exude positivity even when it doesn't feel that way inside. Your mind will catch up when you connect more to your body. If you are reading this and your children have already started to repeat your patterns, bring them on the journey with you. Explain that you are going to end the body bashing and want them to join, too.

SMASH THE SCALE

When I worked in the eating disorder clinic, we would have scale-smashing ceremonies to release anger toward how negative body image held someone back. Appearance is concrete: I have brown hair and brown eyes. Body image is how you feel, your attitude toward your body, and how you think others perceive you. If you suffer from negative thoughts or feelings toward your body, I invite you to smash the scale with your children. (For safety reasons, cover the scale with a blanket and grab some goggles, but otherwise, have some fun!) Let the kids join in. When I smashed the scale with my daughter, I explained to her that the scale wasn't important. Knowing how food and exercise makes me feel is what's important. When we were done, she said, "I am not skinny. I am not fat. I am Claire." I was so inspired, I repeated the same: "I am not skinny. I am not fat. I am Karen."

BE MINDFUL

Be mindful of your body talk. Write down things you say to yourself for a day. Is this an area you need to work on? Do it out loud. Give yourself a compliment out loud. Anytime I give a compliment to one of my kids, I set an intention to also give myself one. Then I ask them to do the same. Part of giving is receiving. They are not separate. You can't have one without the other. As you work to untangle your self-worth from how your body looks, practice the gift of positive self-talk out loud as well as inside.

After you take a mental note of how you speak to yourself about your body, bring in the awareness of actions you take or don't take because of negative body image:

- Are you moody if you judge how you ate?
- Do you hide your body when you change?
- Do you avoid wearing a bathing suit without a cover up?
- Do you ever walk around in your underwear?
- Do you lean into a hug or pull back when someone gets too close?
- Do you avoid shorts or certain clothes because you judge parts of your body?

Getting comfortable with the uncomfortable will go a long way in showing your children how to be comfortable in their own skin. Discussions are important, but actions will deepen the practice and result in change. Look at your body in the mirror and fully take it in without hiding yourself. Give yourself a massage as you put lotion on after a shower. Connecting with your body will allow you to see yourself differently. What we give attention to blossoms, but what we avoid gets weaker. If you begin to avoid taking action or confronting your feelings, return to the letter in the exercise at the end of this chapter. Remember the legacy you want to leave your children and the strength you want them to have for future generations. Let them truly see and feel your worth of yourself so they too can feel worthy.

WORKSHEET: A LETTER TO MY CHILDREN

I wrote this letter to my children, and I invite you to write one in the space below.

To My Clairebear and Lion,

From the moment I first held you in my arms, something changed for me. All the excuses, ways I held myself back, or times I thought I was stuck went away. I knew I needed to be braver and face my internal struggles so you knew that was a strength and something to strive for. You see, while I am here to raise you the best way I know how, you gave me the courage to live my best life. How could I say you deserved true happiness and inner peace without knowing I did as well. I have struggled with feeling depressed, with feeling anxious, with low self-esteem, and making unhealthy choices. We all do. So will you. Those struggles are to be embraced, not hidden. This I have learned. They help us heal and others heal when we share. So I set out on a mission to put this content into the world so that if you ever struggle, you know asking for help and showing up is the way out. And so, when you were born, I made a promise to you.

I promise to fill your world with so much love that you always have a safe place to return to when things feel tough. I promise to not soothe your frustration, sadness, or anger no matter how much I want to wave them away for you, but to teach you how to handle and channel those emotions so they won't rule your world in a negative way. I promise to never take the easy road and to go after everything I want in life so you know it is possible for you. I promise to trust you when it is time to fly from the nest and to support your choices even if they hurt me.

I promise to show you how to be comfortable in your own skin and to quiet the inner voice that may tell you that you are not enough. I promise not to think I am always right and to listen to what you have to say, because it is clear you are already wise beyond your years. I promise to take lots of pictures and be in most of them so you have memories to make you smile, whether I feel pretty that day or not. I promise to always be an honest, real, and peaceful presence in your life. I promise, when you make mistakes, I will not shame you but guide you to let them teach you to grow into the person you are meant to be. I promise to go after my entire bucket list so you can see that a woman can be an amazing mother and still be personally fulfilled. I promise to be your rock because you are mine.

And so I ask you, what is it you want to do with your one wild and precious life? I look forward to a life of supporting you in living it your way.

All my love,
Mama

Your letter:

....

....

....

....

....

....

....

....

....

Conclusion

The key message I want you to take away from this book is this: focus on what you can control. We can control our lifestyle, loving ourselves, and feeling satisfied. We can control creating a positive environment for ourselves and our families. We can't control our bodies being sized or shaped a certain way.

Set boundaries and protect your needs. In order to love your family and everyone around you, you need to love yourself first. Establish a food-neutral home where kids can be raised to have a healthy relationship with food. We want our kids to know who they are on the inside and that it's equally important for them to talk about their bodies and love who they are on the outside.

This book is meant to be a resource you can return to at any time. If you're struggling, you can use it as a reminder that nobody has a perfect relationship with food or their body. Developing these relationships is part of the journey of life, and it's totally normal to feel down about yourself or your choices on occasion.

IF YOU NEED MORE HELP

If reading this book has signaled to you that there are shifts you want to make that are beyond the scope of applying the principles it contains on your own, seek out professional help. Find someone locally who resonates with you. As I mentioned in the last chapter, shame grows in secrecy. We're not meant to do this alone.

Remember, when choosing a local practitioner, you get to be your own healthcare advocate. You have options. Trust your instincts. Here are some questions to consider:

1. "Do you have a specialty in eating disorders? For how long?"
2. "What is your opinion on intuitive eating?"
3. "Have you read the book *Health at Every Size*? Do you practice this philosophy?"
4. (If it is for your child) "How involved are parents, and how are they involved?"

Some practitioners may meet with children alone and then parents are brought in at the end. I have seen other practitioners work only with the child and not include parents at all. Personally, I always involved the parents if the child was living at home, financially dependent, and still in school. Once they turned eighteen, I needed consent from the child to involve the parents, but I always explained the importance of keeping the communication open.

When meeting with a practitioner, engage in a dialogue. Give yourself the power to find someone whose beliefs align with your mission, and trust your intuition. How do you like the conversations with this practitioner, and do you like their answers? Overall, is it a good fit? This is an important step, and you deserve to have the right fit and the right help.

You can always check the National Eating Disorders Association (NEDA) website (https://www.nationaleatingdisorders.org/) to see who is listed as an expert. Interview everyone, even if it is a referral. Not everyone is a good fit.

I began online work in 2015. While I do not provide nutritional therapy or work with an active eating disorder diagnosis, I find so many women struggle with yo-yo dieting, emotional eating, and binge eating. Food and weight take up an excessive amount of their thoughts and energy. The first client I worked with online lost eighty pounds by transforming her mindset with food and freeing herself from the power food had in her life. Since then, I have gone on to work with hundreds of women. I'm currently building a community of women who want to heal, free themselves, and use their newfound confidence to end this legacy of battling with food for the next generation.

You can find more support beyond this book at www.the-freelife.com. There, you can grab our *Chaos to Calm: Survival Guide to a Break Free from Binge Eating*. Also consider subscribing to *The Free Life podcast with Karen Diaz* on iTunes. Sign up for Alexa debriefings on Amazon with *The Free Life with Karen Diaz*.

I can't wait to welcome you as a change maker committed to doing the work within yourself and beyond yourself.

Acknowledgments

In January 2018, my husband, Julio, encouraged me to stop delaying this book and finally put it out there. It would not be here without that loving nudge, and I will never forget.

I am deeply thankful to my parents, Wayne and Mary, for their loving support and belief in me to accomplish my dreams. Without them, I would not be where I am today.

Thank you to my sister, Kristen, one of the most amazing mothers I know. Your endless support knows no bounds, and I am so lucky to have you in my life.

Life is not fun without all of my girlfriends over the years. From Boston to Wyckoff, New Jersey, to Oceanport, New Jersey, to Lakewood Ranch, Florida, or wherever you live—you know who you are. You light me up, pick me up, and I love you for it.

I have so much gratitude for my photographer, Wendy Yalom, who helped bring my vision for the cover to life. Your talent and heart are unmatched. Every time I look at the cover, I will remember you, our day in Miami, and how special you made my daughter, Claire, feel.

I want to extend gratitude and appreciation for the amazing team at Scribe Media for their encouragement, guidance, and passion to make this project come to life in a way that is better than I could have dreamed. Katherine Sears, Rachel Keranen, Nikki Katz, and everyone else who made some imprint into this book. None of your work and support goes unnoticed. Thank you for everything.

Thank you to all my mentors and friends at the Renfrew Center—Page Miliotis, Kathleen Fetter, Esther Gregory, Pam Brodie, Janet Negrini, Alyssa Matthews, Marge Grossman, and all the other women who taught me so much about teamwork and support in the field of eating disorders.

I will never forget the clients I worked with. I remember each and every one of you. Your bravery and courage to show up with an open heart, despite the pain and struggle, has inspired me every step of my life. I will never take for granted how precious of a gift it was to be witness to your transformations. Keep shining.

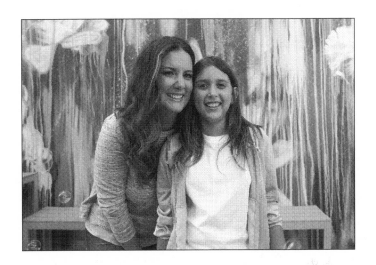

About the Author

KAREN DIAZ is a registered dietitian certified in intuitive eating who helps women overcome eating and body image struggles. She earned her bachelor of science in dietetics from James Madison University and completed her dietetic internship at NewYork–Presbyterian Hospital's Cornell Campus. After graduating, Karen gained experience in pediatrics, food allergies, and weight management both at UMDNJ University Hospital and the research department at Mount Sinai Hospital in New York City. She also worked at the Renfrew Center. Currently she assists women through her signature program, Break Free, which you can learn more about at TheFreeLife.com.